FAT FREE, FLAVOR FULL

Dr. Gabe Mirkin's Guide to Losing Weight and Living Longer

Gabe Mirkin, M.D., and Diana Rich

Little, Brown and Company

Boston ♦ New York ♦ Toronto ♦ London

ALSO BY GABE MIRKIN, M.D.

The Sportsmedicine Book (with Marshall Hoffman)

Getting Thin

FIRST PAPERBACK EDITION

LIBRARY OF CONGRESS CATALOGING-IN-PUBLICATION DATA

Mirkin, Gabe.
    Fat free, flavor full : Dr. Gabe Mirkin's guide to losing weight
and living longer / Gabe Mirkin and Diana Rich. — 1st ed.
        p. cm.
    Includes index.
    ISBN 0-316-57440-6 (hc)
    ISBN 0-316-57473-2 (pb)
    1. Low-fat diet. 2. Low-fat diet — Recipes. 3. Nutrition.
4. Health. I. Rich, Diana. II. Title.
RM237.7.M55 1995
613.2′5 — dc20   94-37919

10 9 8 7 6 5 4

MV-NY

DESIGNED BY JEANNE ABBOUD

*Published simultaneously in Canada by Little, Brown & Company
(Canada) Limited*

PRINTED IN THE UNITED STATES OF AMERICA

Contents

We dedicate this book to Vera Mirkin, who has inspired us with her great spirit and longevity; to Diana's children, Peter, Matthew, Amy and Chris, and Gabe's children, Gene, Jan, Jill, Geoff and Kenny, who may someday learn to like low-fat food.

FAT FREE, FLAVOR FULL

Introduction

Americans eat too much fat.

That's not news. Dozens of cookbooks, magazine articles and health programs tell you how to cut a *little* fat out of your diet. But if you want to lose weight or reverse heart disease without taking drugs, restricting fat only a little is not enough. You need to **restrict fat severely and eat mostly fruits, vegetables, whole grains and beans.**

This book will show you how you can help prevent heart attacks, diabetes, high blood pressure, some types of cancers and many other medical problems by eating no more than **twenty grams of fat per day.** It's the single most important change you can make for better health and a longer life.

I talk to hundreds of people on my radio shows and in my medical practice, and most of them are very confused about what they should or shouldn't do about their diet. It seems that every time you pick up a magazine or newspaper, or turn on the TV or radio, there's a new story about some food or chemical or pill or supplement that is supposed to make you healthier or that you should avoid at all costs. Going to the grocery store has become a frightening experience for many Americans who simply don't know what to believe.

I hope this book will help you understand that most of these stories are circulated by someone who wants to sell you something. You shouldn't have to worry about every bite of food you put in your mouth. You don't need to carry a calculator or a chemistry book when you buy food or sit down to eat. You don't need to worry about all the different types of fats or the amounts of vitamins, minerals, salt, sugar or preservatives in any specific food.

You *do* need to know that there are no magical substances, no special foods or supplements or vitamin pills that will turn a bad diet into a good diet. A healthy diet includes lots of fruits, vegetables, whole grains and beans. It's that simple.

Above all, you *do* need to be concerned if you are eating more food than your body needs. If you are overweight or have a high cholesterol, if you are adding a few pounds every year, or if you go on and off diets to control your weight, you are eating more food than your body can burn up. On the other hand, if you never gain any weight and your cholesterol level is normal, you probably don't need this book. You should thank your parents for your good genes. Most of us are not so lucky.

Blame Your Parents — Then Change Your Life

When you put too much fuel in your car, the extra gasoline spills out onto the pavement. Our bodies don't work that way. If we feed ourselves more fuel than we burn, we store the excess to use later. Some people store fat more efficiently than others.

When food is scarce, people who store fat efficiently live the longest because they need less food to stay alive. If you accept the theory of survival of the fittest, it's easy to understand why most of us have ancestors who stored fat easily. Unfortunately, the genes that may have given your ancestors their advantage in hard times can be a great disadvantage when food is plentiful.

If you inherited the traits that cause you to store fat easily and you eat the average American diet, you accumulate lots of extra fat in your body. Extra fat causes all kinds of problems. If your genes cause you to store the extra fat as plaques in your arteries, you may be very skinny but at great risk for a heart attack. If your genes cause you to store fat primarily in your belly, you are likely to deposit plaques in your arteries as well. If your genes cause you to store fat around your hips and thighs, you are less likely to have plaques in your arteries but you are more at risk for certain types of cancers.

It's easy to see excess fat on your hips or your belly, but to know if you store too much fat in your bloodstream, you have to get blood tests of your cholesterol levels. Many people find cholesterol tests confusing because everyone has both good and bad cholesterol. I'll explain the different kinds of cholesterol in Chapter 3, but for now, it may help to think of "high cholesterol" as medical jargon for too much fat in the bloodstream. Just like excess weight, the problem is caused by taking in more fuel than you burn.

Blaming your parents for the way you store fat may make you feel better, but it won't make you healthier. The good news is that you can transform your body and turn your life around with some simple changes in what you eat and how you exercise. I'll show you how to:

- Give your body less fuel to burn, without ever feeling hungry — by restricting fat severely and eating lots of foods that are high in fiber
- Burn more fuel — by increasing your metabolism with as little as ninety minutes of exercise per week

Our multibillion-dollar weight loss industry thrives because most people believe that the way to lose weight is to go on a diet that limits you to 1,200, 1,000 or even fewer calories a day. These diets ask you to eat tiny portions of food or replace regular food with special diet drinks or foods. You are supposed to use your "will power" and ignore your body's normal signals that tell you when to eat. What these programs don't tell you is that **any diet that leaves you hungry is doomed to failure.** When you feel hungry, your brain signals your body to slow down your metabolism because it thinks you are starving and need to conserve energy. You may lose some weight at first, but you won't go to bed hungry for the rest of your life. As soon as you return to your old eating habits, you quickly gain back any weight you have lost. **My low-fat diet works because you never need to go hungry,** even though you are taking in far fewer calories.

Many people are reluctant to try a low-fat diet because their favorite foods are the ones that are full of fat. In this book, I will help you understand **why** it is so important to change your eating habits and **how** to make truly low-fat food taste delicious. I'll also show you how to start and stay on an exercise program you will love. These may be sweeping changes for you, but they're not hard! You don't need a professional chef or a personal trainer to help you; you can do it all yourself.

My ideas about diet and exercise weren't developed in an ivory tower. I'm a practicing physician who has seen dozens of patients every day for thirty years, and I've talked to thousands of "real people" on my daily radio shows. What's more, I've tested all my theories on my own body. Before I show you how you can change *your* lifestyle, let me tell you about my own battle to control my own cholesterol and how I've kept it down without medication for the past fifteen years. If I can do it, I know you can, too.

CHAPTER 1

My Story

I led my class in cholesterol. I was in my first year of medical school, 22 years old, healthy, and skinny as a rail. Yet a routine blood test showed that my cholesterol count was higher than that of most 50-year-olds with heart disease. I'm one of the people who store all the extra food they eat as fat in their bloodstream. I don't gain weight, but my cholesterol shoots up, depositing plaques in my arteries and setting me up for a heart attack. I was sure that I was doomed to die at an early age. The day I learned that my cholesterol was over 300, I began a lifelong campaign to lower it and keep it down.

Drugs Won't Do It

Thirty-five years ago, medical students were taught that drugs were the only way to lower cholesterol. I started taking a new drug called MER-29, one of the first approved drugs that keep the body from manufacturing cholesterol. After a few months on the drug, I read in a medical journal that many people using it developed cataracts. I stopped taking it immediately, and a short time later it was withdrawn from the market. We have better drugs today, but they all can have unpleasant side effects like itching and muscle aches. I knew there had to be a better way.

Just Exercising Won't Do It

I thought I could outrun my problem with lots of exercise. I enjoyed running, so I embarked on a brutal program of working out three times a day and running more than 100 miles a week. I competed in marathons and other long-distance races throughout the country. All that effort didn't lower my cholesterol enough to protect me from a heart attack. After more than ten years of racing, it had dropped only to 240. A few years ago, scientists proved what I had learned the hard way. Researchers at Grand Forks Human Nutrition Research Center in North Dakota fed a very high fat diet to competitive bicycle racers who were riding more than 300 miles a week. Even though they were burning huge amounts of calories, exercise alone didn't protect them and their cholesterol levels shot up sky high.[1]

Substituting Chicken for Meat Won't Do It

When I figured out that exercise wasn't enough, I decided to see if changing my eating habits would help. Research had shown that saturated fat was the most important single dietary factor in raising cholesterol, so I stopped eating red meat. I ate lots of chicken and turkey instead. My cholesterol didn't drop one point. Many of my patients make the same mistake. They think that on a low-fat diet, you can eat all the chicken you want. Don't believe the propaganda put out by the poultry industry; chicken and turkey have lots of saturated fat, cholesterol and calories.

Eliminating Just Saturated Fat Won't Do It

Then I gave up all sources of saturated fat, such as chicken, whole milk and eggs, but I continued to eat lots of **other** fats, such as margarine. Remember those advertisements on television that told us eating margarine prevents heart attacks? The Food and Drug Administration stopped them because they were deceptive. Margarine contains less saturated fat than butter, so if you substitute margarine for butter, you may lower your cholesterol a little bit (as long as you don't change your total intake of calories). What the ads didn't tell us is that if you substitute air for butter or margarine, you can lower your cholesterol a lot. I didn't understand that, and my cholesterol stayed high.

Meanwhile, my excessive running program meant I had to learn something else about my body — how to deal with injuries from exercise. I had them all. I taught a college course on sports injuries, and that led me to write *The Sportsmedicine Book*.[2] The book sold almost a million copies and was syndicated by the *New York Times*. Soon the CBS radio news service asked me to serve as their fitness commentator. Bob Sherman, a radio station manager, heard my short spots on CBS and invited me to host a daily call-in radio show. That was in 1978, and I began talking to dozens of callers each day about their fitness and health concerns. Many of my callers were as worried about diet and cholesterol as I was, but I still didn't have a good answer for them or for myself.

Pasta and Bread Won't Do It

I was trying to cut down on fat, but I ate a lot of bread and like every other marathon runner, I was eating a heck of a lot of pasta. Bread and pasta are low in fat, but they are also very low in fiber, so it takes a large amount to fill you up. I didn't realize that even though I had cut back on fat, I was still getting lots of extra calories that were converted to fat by my liver.

Reducing All Fats Severely *Will* Do It

By then, Nathan Pritikin was touring the country claiming that the way to prevent heart attacks was to restrict all fats severely. He denounced the American Heart Association's diet as ineffective because it recommended only moderate fat reduction. The man who was called a quack by some members of the medical community was really a prophet with extraordinary insight.

Nathan was a guest on my radio show several times, and I asked him a lot of tough questions — particularly whether his diet would cause mineral deficiencies, as some researchers claimed. Later studies showed that he was right and they were wrong. He also told me I wasn't on a truly low-fat diet. He said that a true low-fat diet means that you avoid all meat, including poultry; all dairy products except skim milk; most bakery products; and *everything* made with any kind of fats or oils.

You Need *Fiber* to Do It

I tried to follow Nathan's advice, but when I took all of the fatty foods out of my diet, there wasn't much left. I was hungry all the time. I work long hours and need to be able to concentrate very hard, so there was no way I could stand constant hunger pangs. I found out why overweight people who go on restricted-calorie diets with tiny portions of food soon return to their old eating habits and regain any weight they have lost. Nobody will go to bed hungry night after night when there is plenty of food around.

The answer came to me in the form of fiber. When I ate lots of fruits, vegetables, whole grains and beans, I felt full and satisfied. These low-fat foods are loaded with fiber, which filled me up and added no calories. Fiber tricks your brain into thinking you have had plenty to eat.

Once I had solved the hunger-pang problem, I knew I was on to something. I started recommending my diet to patients who needed to lose weight as well as to those with cholesterol problems. It worked so well for them that I began to explain my ideas about eating on my radio show. A few months later my listeners started deluging me with their success stories, and I've been hearing them ever since.

Cookies Will Undo It

After I got my cholesterol down where I wanted it, I got cocky and decided it wouldn't hurt to eat a few cookies each night while I worked at my computer. Up went my cholesterol. Could I have maintained my low cholesterol if I had eaten only one or two cookies instead of twenty? Maybe, but most people who set out to cheat a little bit end up cheating a lot. As the potato chip commercial says, "Bet you can't eat just one." I know that if I have fatty foods around, I will eat them. I learned the hard way that I have to keep all temptation out of my house.

You Need Flavor, Too

I still had one big problem. My cholesterol was way down, but I knew I couldn't stick to my new eating habits forever if the food was tasteless and boring. I'm no cook, and I didn't have the foggiest idea how to make beans, vegetables or whole grains taste good. I asked the subscribers to my monthly newsletter, *The Mirkin Report,* to send me their best fat-free recipes. My patients and listeners helped, too, and gradually I built up a collection of ideas for making low-fat food interesting.

When Diana Rich entered my life, she took my dietary requirements as a challenge to her cooking expertise and introduced me to an incredible array of new taste treats. She helped me explore the many ethnic cuisines that are traditionally based on vegetables, beans and grains, with bold seasonings and wonderful textures. Her methods of planning, shopping and stocking the kitchen make low-fat meal preparation a breeze, even for people with busy careers and lots of other responsibilities. You'll read a lot of her cooking tips and recipes in this book.

My cholesterol dropped into the 150s. Now I snack on oranges, apples or grapes whenever I get hungry, and at meals I eat as much of my delicious bean-vegetable-grain dishes as I want. I never feel deprived, and I've kept my cholesterol down for fifteen years.

I've found that if I follow my low-fat diet for almost all of my meals, I can eat out once in a while and my cholesterol doesn't go up. I call it my **19 Meals for Dr. Gabe rule,** and my patients tell me it makes the difference between success and failure. You'll read more about it in Chapter 9.

Why Don't Other Doctors Do It?

Most doctors think that their patients will not stick to diets that restrict fat severely. That tells me that most doctors don't have any idea how to instruct their patients about low-fat diets. It's easier for them to prescribe drugs.

My patients, my listeners and I have stayed on my low-fat diet for years for two reasons:

- I know how to make low-fat food taste good
- I never have to leave the table feeling hungry or go to bed hungry

Just as important, my low-fat diet is easy. You don't have to count calories, figure percentages or keep diaries. And it's cheap — no supplements or formulas to buy, no membership fees. Your grocery bill will be a lot lower when you buy fruits, vegetables, whole grains and beans instead of expensive meats and fatty prepared foods.

My 300-pound cousin asked me how he could lose weight, so I told him about my low-fat diet and gave him my favorite recipe for eggplant-tomato-bean casserole. I explained that I always make a huge batch and then freeze it in fifty individual meal-size microwave dishes. He set out to follow my diet. When I saw him a few weeks later, I asked him how he was doing. He replied that he wasn't doing very well. The casserole tasted so good that he ate all fifty servings at one sitting.

It's All in Learning *How* to Do It

My low-fat diet is a permanent change in lifestyle, not a short-term fix. If you are like most people, you will need to learn new ways to plan and cook low-fat meals that taste good. You probably also could use some ideas for enjoyable exercise that doesn't take much time or defeat you with injuries.

That's why I wrote this book. The next six chapters explain why it's so important for you to change your lifestyle, and debunk a lot of the myths and misinformation about diet and nutrition. If you want to get right into How to Do It, turn to Chapters 8 to 11. They tell you how to get started, how to make food taste good and how to get the most from your exercise program in as little as ninety minutes a week. Chapter 12 has answers to the questions I get asked most often on my radio show, and Chapter 13 has 275 great recipes to help you get started on your new fat-free, flavor-full lifestyle. Turn the pages and I'll teach you how.

CHAPTER 2

What's Wrong with Fat?

Most Americans eat too much. Consuming too many calories causes or contributes to many of our most serious diseases and health problems.

We eat more calories than we need because there is too much fat in our diets. The *average* American eats a whopping **85 grams of fat per day.** *You* may be taking in even more than that.

What's Wrong with Fat?

- **Fat has far more calories than any other food.** Gram for gram, fat has more than twice as many calories as carbohydrates, sugars or proteins. Fats have 9 calories per gram. Carbohydrates and proteins have 4. An 8-ounce baked potato has 129 calories, while 8 ounces of potato chips have 1,200. A cup of skim milk has 97 calories, but a cup of ice cream has 350.

- **Fat makes foods taste so good that we eat too much.** It's the feel of fat in our mouth that we love. Fat makes ice cream smooth. It makes sauces thick and velvety. Fat can be heated to much higher temperatures than water, so food cooked in fat can be seductively crispy and hard to resist — like French fries or potato chips. Most fatty foods don't have much fiber in them, so they don't fill you up. You eat a lot before you feel satisfied and take in loads of extra calories.

- **The fat you eat is easily converted to body fat.** When you eat more food than your body needs, your liver converts the extra calories to fat, regardless of whether the extra food was fat, protein or carbohydrate. It takes extra energy to power the chemical reactions that convert food to body fat. When dietary protein or carbohydrate is converted to body fat, up to 30 percent of the calories is lost as energy. But when the fat you eat is converted to body fat, less than 5 percent of the calories is lost as energy.[3] When you eat 100 extra calories of carbohydrates or proteins, 70 calories end up as body fat. When you eat 100 calories of extra fat, 95 calories end up as body fat.

◆ **Excess body fat causes diseases and keeps you from feeling and looking your best.** That's the bottom line.

Many doctors do not help their patients understand the direct connection between fat and disease. They may give you medication to lower a high cholesterol because it's easier than explaining and monitoring severe fat restriction. If you're like most people, you don't realize that adult diabetes is a disease of fat metabolism, not of sugar metabolism. And you may still believe that high blood pressure is controlled by reducing salt intake, when the most effective treatment by far is reducing fat. Heart disease, diabetes and high blood pressure are serious conditions that can be **reversed** with low-fat eating and exercise, often without any additional medication.

If you weigh more than you did ten years ago, if you are adding a pound or two (or more) each year, or if you keep your weight stable by going on crash diets and then regaining the weight (yo-yo-ing), you are consuming more calories than your body needs. You may already be suffering from heart disease, high blood pressure or diabetes, or perhaps getting warning signals, or you may have a family history of these diseases or of certain types of cancers (see Table 1, page 14).

People who have warning signals or diseases of Western civilization that are linked to high fat intake should restrict their intake of fat to fewer than 20 grams of fat each day. Nobody really knows how much fat you can eat safely if you are **not** overweight or at increased risk for developing a heart attack or cancer. However, we do know that 85 grams of fat each day is too much.

Why 20 Grams of Fat?

If you are of average height and activity level, you need about 1,800–2,500 calories per day to meet your energy needs. If you take in more than that, you are giving your body extra fuel that it doesn't need, so it gets

Table 1. Risk Factors for Common Diseases

Heart Attack Risk Factors	Breast Cancer Risk Factors
Smoking	Family history of breast cancer
Obesity	High-fat diet
High-fat diet	Late menopause
Abnormal cholesterol levels	Early onset of menstruation
Family history of heart attacks	Late first pregnancy
Family history of abnormal cholesterol	No breastfeeding
Chest pain	
High blood pressure	
Prostate Cancer Risk Factors	*Diabetes Risk Factors*
Family history of prostate cancer	Family history of diabetes
High-fat diet	Obesity
Exposure to human wart virus	High-fat diet
Numerous partners	

If any of these risk factors apply to you, you should be on a low-fat diet.

stored as fat. When you eat 85 grams of fat, that's 765 of your calories for the day. You would have to eat tiny portions of every other kind of food to end up with your 1,800–2,500 total. Since you're a normal person who eats when you're hungry, you end up eating more than your body needs and the excess accumulates day by day.

When you limit your fat to 20 grams per day, you get 180 calories from fat — only 7 to 10 percent of your total calorie needs. With all the rest, you can eat lots of high-fiber foods — fruits, vegetables, beans and whole grains — and feel full and satisfied without taking in more fuel than your body needs.

This may sound like calorie counting, but I would never ask you to count the calories you eat each day. I know that never works. Even if you think you can use will power and leave the table hungry after every meal, your brain will think you are starving and slow your metabolism down so you burn fewer calories. That doesn't happen when you cut your fat intake down to 20 grams a day. You never have to feel hungry. All the filling, high-fiber foods you eat trick your brain into thinking you haven't changed anything, so it doesn't put your body into starvation mode.

Low-Fat Fundamentals

When you switch to my low-fat diet, you will eat:

- Very little fat
- Lots of fiber
- Lots of antioxidant vitamins and other phytochemicals

In Chapter 8, I'll give you a complete explanation of the foods to eat and the ones to avoid. Here are the basics:

Very little fat. On my low-fat diet, you eat lots of fruits, vegetables, whole grains and beans. You can have as much of these foods as you want to feel comfortably full and satisfied. You never need to be hungry. You do not need to measure portions or limit yourself to a certain number of servings per day. These foods are full of fiber, which fills you up without adding a lot of calories.

You can also eat low-fat foods that don't contain fiber, but you can't eat them in unlimited amounts. These foods include skim milk and yogurt made from skim milk; fish and shellfish; fat-free breads and pasta made from refined flour; and sugar and other fat-free sweets. You can have five servings of these foods a day. You should include at least one cup of skim milk or yogurt each day, and have three or four servings of seafood a week.

All foods — even a grape or a stalk of celery — have some fat, so to stay under 20 grams per day you need to avoid foods that have more than 2 grams of fat per serving. That means no meat, no chicken or turkey, no eggs or whole-milk dairy products; no bakery products except fat-free breads; no butter, margarine or oils; no nuts or seeds; and no fried foods or other prepared foods made with fats.

If you follow these guidelines for 19 out of your 21 meals each week, you can eat any foods you want (in moderation) at 1 or 2 meals. That's the 19 Meals for Dr. Gabe rule (see page 82), which makes it easy to stay on my low-fat diet forever.

Lots of fiber. Fiber is the part of food that is not absorbed and passes undigested through your body. It makes you feel full, so you consume fewer calories. The foods that are lowest in fat are usually highest in fiber: fruits, vegetables, whole grains and beans.

Fiber lowers cholesterol by binding to bile acids, the building blocks that your liver uses to make cholesterol. A team of physicians in Lexington, Kentucky, showed that lowering fat consumption lowers cholesterol. However, when you add lots of fiber to a low-fat diet, you lower cholesterol even more.[4] Fiber also draws water to your stool, increasing bulk and preventing constipation.

Most people don't eat nearly enough fiber. There's very little fiber in the all-American diet of hamburgers, pizza, fried chicken and beer. Foods made from animal products never have any plant fiber, and processed foods made with vegetables and fruits frequently have most of the fiber removed. Baked potatoes, apples and oranges contain many times more fiber than potato chips, apple jelly or orange juice.

You need at least 35 grams of fiber per day to lower cholesterol significantly, and the average American gets only 11 grams. Nature isn't the cause; our culture and our taste buds are. A serving of unrefined brown rice contains 5.5 grams of fiber. Refining rice removes 87 percent of the fiber, and a serving of white rice contains only 0.7 gram. White bread isn't any bargain, either. It contains only half a gram of fiber per slice, compared to whole-grain breads which contain 7 times as much, or 3.5 grams of fiber. When only the wealthy class could afford white flour, white bread became a status symbol. Dark breads and whole grains were peasant foods. Now most people buy refined foods, so that's what manufacturers provide.

When you go on a low-fat, high-fiber diet, you will eat fruits instead of their juices, whole grains in place of white rice, pasta or white bread, whole-grain cereals instead of refined ones and beans instead of meat and chicken.

Lots of antioxidant vitamins and other phytochemicals. My low-fat diet is loaded with the antioxidant vitamins A, C and E. Vitamins are chemical compounds that the human body needs to grow and function normally. Vitamins A, C and E are called the antioxidant vitamins because one of their important jobs is to prevent certain oxidizing chemical reactions that can be harmful to your body. The antioxidant vitamins help to prevent heart disease because LDL cholesterol must be oxidized before it can form plaques in your arteries. You will read about LDL cholesterol in Chapter 3 and about vitamins and other phytochemicals (plant chemicals) in Chapter 5.

Orange, yellow and green fruits and vegetables have lots of vitamin A; citrus and many other fruits and vegetables contain vitamin C; and just about every kind of food contains vitamin E. As I explain in Chapter 5, you don't need vitamin pills because there is no evidence that large amounts of these vitamins are more protective than small amounts, and some evidence that large doses of vitamins can be harmful. If you eat vitamin pills *instead* of fruits and vegetables, you will miss the hundreds of other phytochemicals found in plants that help to keep you healthy.

Who Should Be on My Low-Fat Diet?

For ten years, I told **Larry J.** that he was a walking time bomb and should be on a low-fat diet. He was a writer who smoked to stay alert and ate tremendous amounts of fatty foods to supply energy to help him work day or night. He had a blood pressure of 150/100, a cholesterol of 280 and chest pains that were severe enough to cause him to seek consultation with a cardiologist. But since his electrocardiograms were normal, Larry didn't feel any need to change his lifestyle. When he had his heart attack, I was the first person called to see him in the emergency room. Now he's on my diet, never felt better and his cholesterol is normal. The heart attack saved his life.

Eating mostly fruits, vegetables, grains and beans is a drastic change from the typical American diet. It's hard to motivate people to make the change unless they are very unhappy with their present situation. Like Larry, you may be scared into action by a heart attack. If you are smarter than he was, you will heed the warning signals before such a life-threatening event.

You should definitely be on a low-fat diet if you have high blood cholesterol or high blood pressure or are overweight; if you have diabetes, chronic constipation or gall bladder disease; or if you are at increased risk for developing a heart attack, diabetes, or cancers of the prostate, breast, uterus, colon or gall bladder (see Table 1). You may **choose** to be on this diet if you want to do all you can to prevent heart attacks and certain types of cancers, or just to look and feel good.

In the next two chapters I will show you how fat causes and aggravates the most common diseases of Western civilization and how you can reverse them with my low-fat lifestyle.

CHAPTER 3

Heart Disease and Fat

Jim K. was 50 when he first called me on my radio show. He had vague chest pains; his father and two brothers had died from heart attacks before age 60. Jim had been evaluated by a cardiologist, who had found no evidence of heart disease and told him not to worry. His cholesterol was 220 and he had a very low good HDL cholesterol of 20. I told him I thought he was in big trouble because his HDL wasn't nearly high enough to cover his 160 LDL, and recommended that he try my low-fat diet and an exercise program. He called me four weeks later to say that he was following the diet and alternating between a stationary bicycle and a rowing machine. He proudly reported that his cholesterol was 180, with a good HDL of 28 and the bad LDL down to 90. Jim called me recently to say that he had just turned 60 and thinks everyone should eat and exercise the way he does.

Almost everyone understands that eating too much food and fat causes heart attacks. Yet many people don't know that the plaques in your arteries can be dissolved just by changing your diet. In 1975, Dr. Robert Wissler of the University of Chicago showed that severe fat restriction and drugs could dissolve plaques in the arteries of monkeys.[5] An article by Dr. Dean Ornish in the British journal *Lancet* reported that arteriosclerotic plaques regressed when people changed the habits that caused the plaques to form in the first place, switching to a diet that contained mostly fruits, vegetables, whole grains, cereals and beans.[6] Dozens of other studies show the same results.

If you've already had a heart attack, you need to start a low-fat diet immediately. You should also make drastic changes if you are getting the warning signs of heart disease or arteriosclerosis.

How to Tell if You're Likely to Have a Heart Attack

A heart attack has two components. First, you lay down fatty plaques in your arteries over the years until eventually the flow of blood slows to a trickle. Second, you suddenly develop a clot that completely blocks the flow of blood to a part of your heart muscle, depriving it of oxygen and causing it to die.

Doctors measure blood cholesterol to predict whether you are likely to lay down plaques. They use another test called Lp(a) to predict susceptibility to forming clots.

When we talk about measuring **cholesterol,** we are actually measuring the different lipoproteins that carry fat in your bloodstream. The chemical cholesterol is just one component of these little balls. The box on pages 20–21 gives a detailed explanation of cholesterol and lipoproteins.

Lots of people — including many doctors — still use the American Heart Association's guideline that a total cholesterol over 200 means you are at risk, and if it is under 200, you are not at risk. Don't believe it. You can be at great risk with a total cholesterol of 150 and no risk with a total of 300. You need to know your cholesterol *fractions.* Your total cholesterol contains both good (Healthy) HDL Cholesterol and bad (Lousy) LDL Cholesterol. These numbers are much more important than your total cholesterol level. You want to have as much of the good HDL cholesterol and as little of the harmful LDL as possible.

LDL and HDL Cholesterol

The Lousy LDL carries cholesterol in your bloodstream onto your artery walls to form plaques. The Healthy HDL carries cholesterol from your bloodstream to your liver, where it is converted to bile and eliminated from your body. People who have high blood levels of the Healthy HDL cholesterol and low blood levels of the Lousy LDL cholesterol are the ones least likely to have heart attacks.

We can predict your risk of having a heart attack by using tables that show how much of the good HDL you need to balance your bad LDL cholesterol. If your LDL is 100, you need to have an HDL of at least 40. If your LDL is 140, your HDL should be at least 70. Table 2 (page 22) will help you check the numbers your doctor gives you.

If your HDL is lower than the number needed to balance your LDL, you should be on a low-fat diet. If your LDL is greater than 140, you are at risk of suffering from a heart attack and should be on a low-fat diet, no matter what amount of HDL you have.

Lipoproteins — LDL, HDL and VLDL

The function of lipoproteins in your body is complicated, but I hope this explanation will help you understand why HDL is Healthful and LDL is Lousy. The most important concept for you to know is how excess fat keeps your body from removing the Lousy LDL.

Fat is carried in your bloodstream in little fatty balls coated with protein, called lipoproteins. There are several different types of lipoprotein balls in your bloodstream: VLDL, LDL and HDL. When you take in more food than you need, your liver converts all of the extra calories to a type of fat called triglyceride. (It doesn't make any difference whether the source of the extra calories is carbohydrate, fat or protein.) Then your intestines and liver take 1,500 triglyceride molecules, combine them with a lesser number of cholesterol molecules and cover them with a protein coat to form a lipoprotein ball called Very Low Density Lipoprotein, or **VLDL** cholesterol.

VLDL travels through your bloodstream, giving up triglyceride molecules continuously as a source of energy for your cells until it contains mostly cholesterol molecules and very few triglyceride molecules. This new ball is called Low Density Lipoprotein, or **LDL** cholesterol, which contains a much higher proportion of cholesterol to triglyceride molecules. LDL cholesterol, by itself, is thought to be harmless. However, if it is oxidized by chemical reactions in your body to form **oxidized LDL,** it can form plaques in arteries that obstruct the flow of blood and cause heart attacks and strokes (Figure 1). Fruits, vegetables and olive oil help to

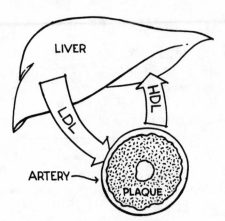

Fig. 1. Lousy LDL carries cholesterol to the arteries and forms plaques.

Healthy HDL carries cholesterol to your liver so it can be eliminated from your body.

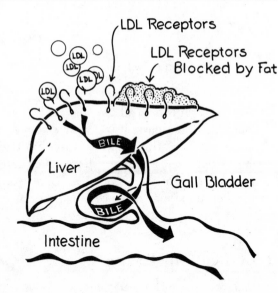

LDL Receptors

LDL Receptors
Blocked by Fat

Liver

Gall Bladder

Intestine

Fig. 2. Your liver has LDL receptors which remove the Lousy LDL from your bloodstream.

If fat clogs your LDL receptors, they can't do their job.

prevent LDL from being converted to oxidized LDL. LDL can also be removed from your bloodstream by little hooks on your liver cells, called LDL receptors, and converted to bile, which can be removed from your body (Figure 2). Eating too much food or too much fat clogs the LDL receptors on your liver cells, so they can't do their job of removing LDL cholesterol from the bloodstream, increasing blood levels of LDL and forming plaques in arteries. Reducing your intake of food or fat increases the number of working LDL receptors, lowers blood levels of LDL and helps to prevent heart attacks.

◆ **Reducing calories causes the liver to make less VLDL cholesterol.**
◆ **Reducing fat causes the liver to remove more LDL cholesterol.**

HDL helps to prevent heart attacks. It is manufactured by various cells throughout the body and carries cholesterol from the bloodstream to the liver, where it can be removed and converted to bile. Unlike LDL cholesterol, it does not require special receptors on liver cells to be removed from the bloodstream. Therefore, a high-fat diet does not **prevent** HDL from being removed by your liver cells, but a very low fat diet increases the rate at which the liver removes HDL from your bloodstream.

John R. had a good HDL of 25 and a bad LDL of 120. From Table 2, we can see that an HDL of 25 will cover only an LDL of 85. John started a strict low-fat diet, and when he returned for a retest one month later, he had lowered his LDL to 75 — through diet alone. He should be able to maintain that level easily just by limiting the amount of fat he eats.

When you start a low-fat diet, you can expect all the changes in your blood cholesterol level to occur within ten days. If you reduce your fat intake and ten days later you do not have the proper relationship between HDL and LDL, try cutting out even more fat. Most people can lower their LDL enough just with stringent fat restriction. Those who cannot get to these ratios with diet alone may also need medication to achieve the results they want.

Some People Need Medication, Too

Susan M. had a heart attack at age 39, which is very unusual because the female hormone, estrogen, helps to protect women from heart attacks. Susan was 5 feet tall and weighed 167 pounds, and her cholesterol was 400 with an HDL of 60 and an LDL of 290. Her doctor placed her on one baby aspirin a day and a heart medication and told her to go on a low-fat diet. After one month, her cholesterol values had not changed and she had not lost weight. She had heard me talk about my low-fat diet on the radio and came to see me to find out why it wasn't working for her.

Susan told me she had not eaten any red meat or butter, but she did eat tuna fish or salmon for lunch and chicken for dinner almost every

Table 2. How Much Healthy HDL Do You Need to Cover Your Lousy LDL?

If your LDL is:	You need an HDL of at least:
90	35
100	45
110	50
120	55
130	60
140	70

If your LDL is over 140, you should be on a low-fat diet regardless of your HDL level.

day. I suggested that she tighten up her low-fat diet by eliminating chicken, eating fish only three times a week and loading up on fruits, vegetables, grains and beans. One month later, her cholesterol was 210 with an HDL of 30 and an LDL of 170. That was a significant drop, but Susan needed lovastatin and niacin to bring her cholesterol down further. She is maintaining normal levels now with the combination of medication and her strict low-fat diet.

Sam T. came to see me for an allergic skin rash. In the course of evaluating him, I found that his cholesterol was 190 with an HDL of 20 and an LDL of 140. Since his father and brother had both had heart attacks, he was at high risk, so I ordered the special blood test called Lp(a). It was high, showing that he had a clotting disorder. This is one condition that cannot be treated by diet alone. Sam needed large doses of niacin to raise his HDL *and* a low-fat diet to lower his LDL. Today, he takes more than 3,500 mg of niacin each day, and his cholesterol is 140 with an HDL of 70 and an LDL of 50.

Some people need both a low-fat diet *and* medication to lower a very high LDL. For people like Susan and Sam, even the most stringent low-fat diet may not be enough. However, diet is an essential part of the treatment. Don't be lulled into thinking that medication can take the place of changing your eating habits.

Surgery Is Not a Permanent Fix

If you are in serious trouble, your doctor may recommend surgery to clear obstructed arteries. Don't be deceived into thinking that surgery will permanently protect you from a heart attack. You need to change your lifestyle or the obstruction will quickly build up again, and you'll be back where you started.

When you have angioplasty, a balloon is inserted into the arteries on the surface of your heart to stretch the arteries and let more blood through. Many people who have this procedure end up with the blockage returning within a few months. Bypass surgery isn't much more effective. The surgeon inserts an artificial artery to reroute blood flow around the obstructed artery. People who have bypass surgery are less likely to suffer a fatal heart attack for the first year, but after that they are no better off than the patients who refused to have surgery.

Unless you change your eating habits, the high-fat diet that caused the blockage in the first place will cause the stretched or replaced arteries to fill up with plaques again. Effective treatment for arteriosclerosis must include a low-fat diet, whether you have surgery or not.

A Low-Fat Diet Lowers HDL Cholesterol in a Good Way

If you go on a low-fat diet, your good HDL cholesterol may go down, but that does not mean you are at increased risk for developing a heart attack. A low-fat diet lowers both the good HDL and bad LDL cholesterol. Both of these changes are healthful. Your liver cells remove HDL and LDL from your bloodstream. A low-fat diet unclogs the LDL receptors on your liver cells so that they can remove both LDL and HDL cholesterol at a faster rate. Think of a bathtub that has a constant water level because the water is running in at the same rate that it is passing out through the drain. If you put in an additional drain, the water runs out faster and the water level drops. The same thing happens when you go on a low-fat diet. Your blood level of HDL cholesterol goes down in a good way because it is removed at a faster rate.

Can a High HDL Harm You?

Women who eat a lot of fat and have a high HDL cholesterol are at low risk of suffering heart attacks, but they are at increased risk for developing breast cancer. A high-fat diet increases a woman's chances of developing breast cancer, and it also raises blood levels of HDL cholesterol. When such women go on low-fat diets, they lower both their HDL and LDL cholesterol levels and reduce their chances of developing breast cancer, as you will read in the next chapter.

Can Your Cholesterol Be Too Low?

> **Dave B.** came to see me because he had read stories in the newspapers about a study that showed that people who have low blood cholesterol levels are more likely to die of cancer. His total cholesterol was 121, with a good HDL cholesterol of 50 and a bad LDL cholesterol of 60. I told him that the data show that people who have cancers often lose their appetites and eat very little, which causes their cholesterol to go down. I told him that his chances of dying of a heart attack are close to zero and his blood cholesterol level is associated with a very long life span. He responded by telling me that his mother is 93 and still plays golf.

An article published in the journal *Circulation* showed that people with low cholesterol levels rarely die of heart attacks, but they are more likely to die of strokes, liver cancer, lung disease, alcoholism and by suicide.[7] This does not mean that a low cholesterol **causes** any of the diseases. It's the other way around: the diseases lower cholesterol.

Having a low cholesterol doesn't cause depression. People who are depressed often lose their appetites, so they eat less and that lowers cholesterol. People who have lung, liver or pancreatic cancer also eat less food than healthy people, and so do alcoholics. Any disease that causes you to eat less will lower cholesterol.

There are weak data to show that a very low cholesterol may thin your blood and possibly increase your chance **slightly** of suffering a stroke, because very thin blood may be more likely to leak through blood vessels and accumulate in tissue. The data show that the risk of stroke is increased from 1 in 10,000 to 2 in 10,000. That's insignificant compared to the fact that people with high cholesterol have more than three times the chances of developing heart attacks as those with lower cholesterol, and more than half of the deaths in this country are associated with heart attacks. Furthermore, the overall death rate of people who have cholesterol under 160 is far less than that for people with cholesterol over 200.[8]

Other Diseases and Fat

Joanne H. came to see me for a high blood pressure of 165/105. She refused to take the drugs that her doctor prescribed because she didn't want to "take anything that isn't natural." Her "natural" approach included eating only special low-salt foods to treat her high blood pressure. I told her that there is no evidence that **low-salt** foods help to lower blood pressure, but there are lots of studies that show a **low-fat** diet lowers high blood pressure. She went on my "natural" low-fat diet, lost a lot of weight and now has a normal blood pressure of 115/75.

High Blood Pressure and Fat

Many doctors still tell their patients with high blood pressure just to stop eating salt. We now know that a low-fat diet lowers high blood pressure far more effectively than a low-salt diet does.

Arteries are like balloons. When your heart contracts, they widen to receive extra blood. This lowers the resistance against the flow of blood and keeps your blood pressure from rising too much. Plaques make your arteries stiff and prevent them from expanding to receive the blood when your heart contracts, so your blood pressure goes up too high. The plaques in arteries that cause high blood pressure are formed from excess fat, as I explained in the last chapter. When you lose excess weight, the plaques dissolve. **Weight loss alone can lower blood pressure to normal** in more than half of the people who have high blood pressure.

Salt holds water in blood vessels, so excess salt can increase blood volume and thus raise your blood pressure a little. However, salt is not the cause of most cases of high blood pressure. When you go on a low-fat diet and begin to dissolve the plaques in your arteries, you are getting at the cause of the problem. When most people with high blood pressure increase their intake of salt, their blood pressure does not rise further. Moderate salt restriction does not help the vast majority of people with high blood pressure. Severe salt restriction can lower blood pressure, but it can also raise blood levels of the harmful LDL cholesterol. Giving diuretics to and restricting salt in people who have high blood pressure can cause a low-salt syndrome characterized by severe muscle weakness.

If you have high blood pressure or swollen feet, you may possibly benefit from not adding **extra** salt to your food and not eating salty-tasting foods. You do not need to seek out special low-salt foods or count milligrams of sodium in your diet. It's far more important for you to stop drinking alcohol, start an exercise program and, of course, start your low-fat diet to lose weight and reverse the buildup of plaques in your arteries.[9]

Diabetes and Fat

> Fredricka S. came to see me for her diabetes, which she developed at age 52. She was taking insulin injections and was 5 feet 7 inches and weighed 220 pounds. Her doctor had already told her that she could probably "cure" her diabetes if she lost weight, but she had failed on every diet she tried. I put her on unlimited fruits, vegetables, grains and beans and not much else and within six months, she weighed 142 pounds, was off all drugs and had normal fasting blood sugar levels.

If you're like most people, you believe that diabetes means you don't have enough insulin and shouldn't eat sugar. For the 90 percent of diabetics who develop their disease after age 50, that's just not true! There are two main causes of diabetes. Either you don't have enough insulin to keep your blood sugar level from rising too high or your cells are unable to respond to insulin. Studies show that diabetes in adults is usually caused by inability to respond to insulin, rather than not having enough insulin.[10] Late-onset diabetes is a **disorder of fat metabolism manifested by high blood sugar levels, not a disorder of sugar metabolism.**

Your risk for diabetes is greatest if your parents had the disease or if you are grossly overweight. Diabetes is the sixth leading cause of death in Americans. It is a miserable disease, causing all kinds of complications, such as heart attacks and nerve damage that can lead to blindness or loss of limbs. If you have diabetes or are at risk of developing it, please read this section carefully so you will understand why a low-fat diet and exercise are so important for you. You can make a huge difference in the quality of your life.

Insulin circulates in your bloodstream and drives sugar from your bloodstream into your cells. Diabetes occurs when insulin does not do its job, permitting sugar to accumulate in your bloodstream.

Each cell in your body is like a balloon full of fluid. On the outside surface of each cell are little hairs called insulin receptors. Insulin cannot drive sugar from your bloodstream into cells until it first attaches to the insulin receptors. When you have excess fat in your diet and excess fat stored in your body, the receptors are pushed inside the cells so insulin can't attach to them. When the amount of fat is reduced, the receptors pop back out and become available to receive insulin again.

Most people who develop diabetes after age 50 have cells that cannot respond adequately to insulin because they do not have enough insulin receptors. The vast majority of these people can **reverse their diabetes by eating a low-fat diet and losing fat from their bodies.** They are able to go off medication and resume a full, normal life. If you are overweight and have diabetes or have a family history of diabetes, you should start a program of low-fat eating and exercise immediately.

> **Vincent T.** called me on the radio to ask what he could do about impotence. He then volunteered that he was 56 years old, had diabetes and high blood pressure and was taking several medications. When I hear this kind of problem, my first questions are: "How tall are you?" and "How much do you weigh?" Vincent was 5 feet 10 inches and 190 pounds. I explained that his impotence could be caused by nerve damage from the diabetes, by plaques in his arteries that were evidenced in his high blood pressure and certainly by the medications he was taking. He was amazed to hear that there was a connection between his impotence and his other health problems. His family doctor had told him it was just a sign of old age. I told him he needed to lose 50 pounds by going on a low-fat diet and starting an exercise program. I bet him $100 to his $1 that if he did, he could get off the medications, control his diabetes and high blood pressure and regain his sexual function. That's $100 I hope I lose.

Cancer and Fat

When you take in more calories than your body needs, the extra calories stimulate tissue to grow. Uncontrolled growth is cancer. That's why people who are overweight are more likely to suffer from several different types of cancers, including cancers of the prostate, breast, colon, gall bladder and uterus. A low-fat, high-fiber diet appears to help to prevent cancer, probably because you take in fewer calories.

Fats are classified by their chemical structures into different types called saturated, polyunsaturated and monounsaturated, as I explain in Chapter 6. Polyunsaturated fats that are found in vegetable oils, such as corn oil margarine, are *more* likely to cause cancer than the saturated fats found in meats. There's a logical explanation. Your body uses a series of chemical reactions to produce energy and grow new tissues. DNA is the genetic material in cells that tells them how to grow. Many of the chemical reactions produce by-products called oxidants that can damage DNA and cause cells to grow uncontrollably. The breakdown of poly-unsaturated fats produces more oxidants than that of the other types of fats. A polyunsaturated fat called linoleic acid has been shown to be a necessary growth factor for tumors.

Breast and Prostate Cancer

Cancer of the breast is the most common cancer in women. Cancer of the prostate is the second most common cancer in men (after lung cancer). Americans who eat a high-fat diet have a very high incidence of both of these cancers.

The Chinese, who eat a low-fat diet, have a very low rate of prostate and breast cancers. Japanese men who eat low-fat diets have a low inci-dence of prostate cancer, but when they move to the United States and start eating the typical high-fat Western diet, they lose that advantage. Native Africans whose diets are low in fat are relatively immune to prostate and breast cancer, but African Americans who eat our typical high-fat diet increase their chances of developing cancer of the prostate or breast by a factor of ten. Eating a lot of meat causes the brain to produce large amounts of prolactin, a hormone produced by the brains of both men and women that stimulates milk production in the breasts. It also stimulates the breast and prostate to grow, and high blood levels of prolactin are associated with an increased risk for developing prostate and breast cancers.

The female hormone, estrogen, causes breast tissue to grow. The most potent estrogen in a woman's body is called estradiol. Women who eat a lot of fat have high blood levels of estradiol. Blood estradiol levels drop significantly just a few weeks after women reduce their intake of fat from 70 grams a day to 30. Researchers believe that American women can reduce their chance of developing breast cancer fivefold by restricting their intake of fat.[11]

You may have read about a study from Harvard in the *Journal of the American Medical Association*[12] that reported incorrectly that low-fat diets are not associated with a decreased risk of developing breast cancer. The authors compared women on diets that contained 37 percent fat with those who were on a minimal fat restriction of 30 percent. A 30 percent fat diet contains 60 grams of fat per day, which can hardly be called a low-fat diet. A low-fat diet should contain no more than 10 percent fat, or about 20 grams per day. If you reduce your intake of fat only slightly, you probably will not reduce your total intake of calories. You will not lower cholesterol significantly, lose weight or reduce your risk of cancer.

Colon and Gall Bladder Cancer

Your liver serves as a strainer that removes waste products from your bloodstream and turns them into bile, which passes along a tube to be stored in an upside-down muscular balloon called the gall bladder (Figure 3). When you eat food, particularly fatty food, your gall bladder contracts and squeezes bile into your intestines, where it mixes with the food and helps to digest it so the food can be absorbed into your bloodstream. Bile can cause cancer. When it is rubbed on the skins of animals, it causes skin cancer. A high-fat diet causes the liver to make more bile. The extra bile passes through the gall bladder to your intestines, increasing your chances of developing cancer of the gall bladder, and to the colon, increasing your chances of developing cancer of the colon.[13]

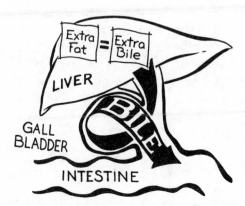

Fig. 3. A high-fat diet causes your liver to make extra bile. Too much bile increases your chances of developing cancer of the gall bladder or colon.

If You Weigh More Than You Like

Mary B. came to see me because she weighed 190 pounds. She was five feet tall and had been on numerous diets for most of her life. She told me that during the course of her dieting, she had lost more than 600 pounds. She would lose weight and gain it right back again because, like most people, Mary couldn't stand to feel hungry all the time. She was delighted to learn that on my low-fat diet, she could eat all the fruits, grains, vegetables and beans she wanted. She lost 15 pounds in the first two months, but after the third month, she seemed to reach a plateau. She wasn't regaining the weight, but she wasn't losing any more, either.

I asked her about her exercise program and she told me she hated to exercise. After I explained the role of exercise in raising metabolism, she grudgingly joined an aerobic dance class for overweight women. She was amazed at how much she enjoyed meeting and working out with the other women in her class. Six years later, she weighs 139 pounds, is still dancing three times a week and has several good friends from her aerobics class.

Even if you do not have any of the health problems or risk factors described in these chapters, excess weight is reason enough to go on a low-fat diet. Few of us are able to carry a 20-pound suitcase very far without getting tired, yet millions of Americans carry the equivalent of one, two or even several suitcases around with them every day. For most people who have a lot of excess weight, it's just a matter of time before they begin to develop other health problems. In the meantime, you probably would like to lose weight just to look better and have more energy.

When I talk about excess weight, I mean excess body fat. Muscles weigh more than fat, so if you are heavy and are all muscle, you're just fine. But if you are a man with more than 12 percent body fat or a woman with more than 22 percent, you're taking in more calories than you need. You can do a quick check with the "inch of pinch" test: pinch the flesh at your waist, on the side of your thigh, and the back of your upper arm between your thumb and forefinger. If there's more than an inch in any of those areas, you probably have too much body fat. You can do a much more accurate measure with a set of fat calipers, which you can obtain by sending $15 to The Mirkin Report, P.O. Box 6608, Silver Spring, Maryland 20916. Many hospitals and clinics also offer simple, inexpensive tests to check body fat content.

Our multibillion-dollar diet industry thrives on all of the people who want to lose weight but don't know how. In the next chapters I'll explain why the old ideas about diet don't work and how you can lose weight **permanently** with my low-fat lifestyle.

CHAPTER 5

Misconceptions about Diet

Prevention magazine surveyed Americans about their eating habits and found that most people don't understand which factors in their diet cause excess weight and disease.[14] Thirty-three percent of all Americans try to avoid food additives, which doesn't make sense. There is no evidence whatever that the additives in the foods that you eat are harmful to your health. The Food and Drug Administration has reviewed all of the food additives in use today and has found them to be safe. Two of the additives, BHA and BHT, have been shown to help prevent cancers.

Forty-three percent of those responding claimed that they try to avoid sugar. This effort is also unfounded. Except for causing cavities, sugar is not harmful. When you eat table sugar, it becomes chemically identical to the sugars found in fruits and other "natural" foods. People who are overweight do not eat more sugar than those who are thin. Sugar consumption has not been linked to heart attacks or cancer.

Fifty percent stated that they try to avoid cholesterol. Cholesterol is found only in foods from animals, such as meat, fish, fowl, dairy products and eggs. It is not found in plants. The amount of cholesterol you *eat* has little to do with the amount of cholesterol *in your bloodstream*. Avoiding a heart attack requires a lot more than just avoiding meat. Potato chips may have no cholesterol, but they are almost pure fat. If you want to lower a high blood cholesterol level, you need to restrict all fats. The evidence is accumulating that vegetarians may be healthier than omnivorous humans, but only if they don't eat a lot of fatty foods.

Common Diet Fallacies

Many of the diets that you may have tried in the past are based on unscientific principles. You can spend a lot of money and suffer a lot of hunger pangs without gaining any long-term benefits.

- **Calorie restriction doesn't work.** You may lose weight, but you will gain it right back when you get tired of going hungry and return to your old eating habits.
- **Restricting just saturated fat** won't work. You need to restrict *all* fats. Chapter 6 explains the different types of fats and sorts out all the conflicting advice you may have heard in the past.
- Don't expect significant benefits from **restricting fat a little bit.** To lose weight or lower cholesterol, you need to restrict fat severely.
- **Avoiding foods that contain cholesterol** will not lower your cholesterol if you continue to eat the same amount of fat.
- **Being a vegetarian** will not help you lose weight or control cholesterol unless you also reduce your intake of fat. Vegetarian meals that include soybeans, vegetable oils, nuts and seeds, eggs and dairy products can be very high in fat.
- You don't need to take **vitamin pills or supplements.** Humans have been on this planet for five million years, and our enzyme systems have not changed suddenly. You can meet all your needs for nutrients with food.
- **No single food is good or bad.** Chapter 7 debunks some of the myths you may have heard about special foods. It's the total amount of food and fat you eat that determines your body fat and cholesterol. I recommend that you avoid some types of foods only because they contain lots of fat.
- Don't be taken in by **fad diets** based on gimmicks. Combining certain foods or supplements and avoiding other combinations will not burn fat or give you any other health benefits.

Calorie-Restriction Diets Don't Work

The multibillion-dollar diet industry offers all sorts of schemes that try to get you to take in fewer calories. Entrepreneurs sell you low-calorie meals and drinks that are supposed to replace food. For example, you may eat a special meal package that contains only 300 calories. As long as you eat this 300-calorie meal four times a day and nothing more, you will lose weight. But your brain and your body will fight you every step of the way.

Your metabolism slows down because your brain thinks you are starving and adjusts your hormones to help you conserve energy. Eventually you will refuse to leave the table hungry after every meal and go to bed hungry every night. When you return to your normal eating habits, you will quickly regain all the weight that you have lost.

If you've tried these methods and failed, don't blame yourself. There is no evidence anywhere that restricting all food causes permanent weight reduction. If the calorie-restriction diet plans had to publicize their failure rates, they would all go out of business.

When you decide to lose weight, it is very important to use a diet that you can follow for the rest of your life. A study in the *New England Journal of Medicine* showed that people who repeatedly lose and gain weight (the "yo-yo" syndrome) are more than twice as likely to suffer heart attacks and premature death as those who have stable weights.[15]

Every time you *lose weight rapidly*, you increase your chances of forming gall stones. Your liver removes many breakdown products of metabolism from your bloodstream and converts them to bile, which passes to and is stored in your gall bladder. Bile contains cholesterol, which tends to form gall stones, and bile acids, which keep the cholesterol soluble so it does not form stones. Bile acids are formed from the food that you eat. When you restrict food, your liver markedly reduces its production of bile acids, causing the cholesterol to form stones.

When you *regain the weight you lost*, your liver manufactures extra fat, which passes into your bloodstream to form plaques in arteries. Plaques block arteries to cause heart attacks. Both animals and humans who yo-yo die younger than those who remain fat.[16] Furthermore, **the weight you lost was both fat and muscle, and what you regain is almost all fat.**

To lose weight permanently, you must be able to eat when you feel hungry. That's why low-fat eating works. A 10 percent reduction in dietary fat will cause a 25 percent reduction in calories. A low-fat diet is really a low-calorie diet, with one important difference: you can stay on it forever. You don't ever have to feel hungry or deprived. You avoid foods that are rich in fat, but you can eat fruits, vegetables, whole grains and beans *whenever you are hungry*, and their fiber makes you feel full.

Reducing Only Saturated Fat Doesn't Work

Doctors used to treat high blood cholesterol levels by recommending that you reduce your intake only of saturated fats. Now they know that if you substitute other fats for saturated fats, you will lower your cholesterol only a little bit and you won't lose any weight at all. A low-saturated-fat diet won't help you lose weight or lower cholesterol significantly because it usually does nothing to reduce your total intake of calories.

Saturated fat raises blood cholesterol more than any other dietary component, but only if you take in too many calories. When you eat exactly the amount of food your body needs, saturated fat is burned for energy and does not accumulate in your body. Taking in fewer calories than your body requires makes your cholesterol go down, even if *most* of the calories are from saturated fat.

Reducing Fat a Little Bit Doesn't Work

If you want to lose weight or lower cholesterol without taking drugs, don't depend on diets that tell you to reduce fat a little. The American Heart Association's Step I diet recommends that Americans reduce their intake of fat from an average 37 percent to 30 percent. If that doesn't lower your cholesterol (and it almost never does), the Step II diet recommends further reductions in fat intake, down to 25 percent. That's still not enough. Articles in the *Journal of Family Practice*, the *Journal of the American Medical Association* and the *British Medical Journal* show that reducing fat intake that little doesn't lower your cholesterol.[17] The AHA's Step III diet takes you down to 20 percent, but a study in the *American Journal of Clinical Nutrition* shows that doesn't work either.[18] The only people who had a significant lowering of their cholesterol on that diet were the ones who restricted fat far more than was recommended and lost a lot of weight. You must get down to 10 percent of your calories from fat, or 20 grams of fat per day, to lower cholesterol significantly.

Many physicians still recommend the AHA Step I, II and III diets because they believe that people won't put up with severe fat restriction. They are wrong. You can stick to a low-fat diet easily if you know how to make the food taste good. This book shows you how.

"No-Cholesterol" Foods Do Little to Lower Your Cholesterol

The Food and Drug Administration now prohibits "no-cholesterol" claims on high-fat foods. Cholesterol is manufactured by all animals, so it is found in meat, chicken, eggs, dairy products, fish, humans, ants, snails, worms and spiders. It is not found in plants. Food producers who used the no-cholesterol label took advantage of people's fear of heart attacks without giving them the information they really need about the dangers of fat. You can be on a no-cholesterol diet by being a complete vegetarian and still have your cholesterol go up if you eat lots of fat-rich foods such as potato chips, nuts and vegetable oils.

Your own liver manufactures more than 80 percent of the cholesterol in your bloodstream. Less than 20 percent of your cholesterol comes from the food that you eat. If you are eating just the amount of food your body needs, your liver keeps the amount of cholesterol in your bloodstream stable. When you eat more cholesterol from animal products, your liver makes less, and when you decrease your intake of cholesterol, your liver makes more to compensate. On the other hand, if you take in more calories than your body needs, all the extra calories are converted by your liver into extra cholesterol and triglycerides. It doesn't matter whether the extra calories come from animal products (with cholesterol) or vegetable products (with no cholesterol).

Vegetarians Should Restrict Fat, Too

Being a vegetarian helps to protect you from heart attacks *only if you also restrict your intake of fatty foods*. Lots of vegetarian foods are loaded with fat. Most soybean products, such as tofu and vegetarian hamburger substitutes, are high-fat foods, as are nuts and seeds. Many vegetarians use a lot of oil when they cook.

If you are on a *low-fat* vegetarian diet and do not eat dairy products or eggs, you may have added protection against heart attacks. Animal protein raises blood cholesterol more than plant protein does. Animal protein contains a higher ratio of the essential amino acids, which slows down the rate at which the bad LDL cholesterol is removed from the bloodstream.[19]

My low-fat diet is almost a vegetarian diet, since you don't eat meat, poultry, butter or eggs. I do encourage you to eat a limited amount of skim milk products and seafood because they supply some essential nutrients and add variety to your diet. If you want to follow a strict vegetarian low-fat diet with no dairy products or fish, you should take vitamin B_{12}, vitamin D and calcium supplements.

Why You Don't Need Pills

Six out of every ten Americans take vitamin pills and mineral supplements because they think they need them to stay healthy. A lousy diet with vitamin pills is still a lousy diet. Vitamin pills have no special benefits over food and have not extended the maximum human life span.

A vitamin is an organic compound that your body needs *in small amounts* for you to be healthy. Most vitamins are parts of enzymes, substances that speed up chemical reactions. They are not changed by the reaction, even though they cause the same reaction to proceed over and over again. Because vitamins *act* on reactions and are not *used up* as part of reactions, they are required only in small quantities.

Vitamins are absorbed into the bloodstream and enter the cells that need them. There the vitamin combines with another chemical, called an apoenzyme, which is synthesized by the cell to form a complete enzyme. There is only a limited amount of apoenzyme inside the cell that is available to combine with the vitamin. Excess vitamins cannot combine with an apoenzyme that is already bound to another vitamin.

Dr. Victor Herbert, of the Bronx Veterans Administration Hospital, compares vitamins in cells to a traffic intersection. Many cars (chemical reactions) pass through the intersection, but only one police officer (vitamin) is necessary to direct traffic. Bringing in many police officers (excess vitamins) won't cause more cars (chemical reactions) to pass through the intersection.

Can Excess Vitamins Harm You?

The vitamin industry uses all kinds of ploys to promote their products, misinterpreting scientific studies and mounting emotional campaigns about consumers' rights. Most doctors have shrugged their shoulders on the theory that even though they're not necessary, extra vitamins won't hurt you. You might be wasting a lot of money, but that's your decision. Now a very well done study from Finland is causing many people to question that conventional wisdom.

For more than fifty years, scientists have believed that beta carotene (vitamin A) helps to prevent cancer. Recently, scientists in Finland followed 30,000 male smokers for ten years, giving some vitamin E supplements, some beta carotene and some a placebo.[20] Those who took the vitamin E had the same rate of lung cancer as those who took no supplements, but those who took the beta carotene had an 18 percent higher incidence of lung cancer. That doesn't mean that beta carotene causes cancer. However, we do know that large amounts of vitamin A can deplete your body of vitamin E, which *can* increase your chances of developing cancer. The important message is that when you take one chemical in pills, you can cause a deficiency of another chemical in your body.

Scientists have extracted hundreds of chemicals from foods and have shown that some appear to prevent cancer, while others are associated with higher rates of certain cancers. However, the studies evaluate chemicals out of foods and do not evaluate the total effects of the foods. The theory of evolution tells us that those whose bodies adapt best to the environment survive and have children with the greatest chance to survive. The human race has been around for five million years, gradually adapting to the environment. For massive doses of vitamins to make us super healthy, the enzyme systems in our bodies would have had to change radically over the last sixty years, the time vitamin pills have been available.

A multibillion-dollar vitamin industry is trying to convince you that *you need* to take pills and supplements. Before you spend your money, I hope you will consider their profit motive. Here are my rebuttals to some of the misinformation that I have seen in publicity campaigns.

Extra vitamin C doesn't lower cholesterol significantly. Vitamin sellers used studies from several medical journals to show that vitamin C lowers cholesterol. The studies reported that in the winter, tissue and blood levels of vitamin C are lower and blood cholesterol levels are higher.[21] This does not prove that low levels of vitamin C raise blood cholesterol levels. In the winter, people eat fewer vitamin C–rich plant foods. Since they take in less vitamin C, their blood levels of that vitamin drop. At the same time, when they eat fewer plant foods they are likely to eat more of other foods, so they increase their intake of meat and dairy products that are loaded with fat, which raises cholesterol. Vitamin C is necessary for the breakdown of cholesterol, but none of these studies shows that large doses of vitamin C offer any more benefit than eating a small amount of fruit every day.

You don't need extra vitamin E. A report in the *American Journal of Clinical Nutrition* showed that low blood levels of vitamin E are associated with an increased chance of dying from a heart attack.[22] That prompted some vitamin pill sellers to claim that a low-fat diet may cause a vitamin E deficiency. Vitamin E is found in virtually all foods, but it is especially plentiful in vegetable oils. It is one of the antioxidant vitamins that prevent harmful breakdown products from unsaturated fat metabolism, called oxidants, from accumulating in your body. However, your body requires only small amounts of vitamin E, and when you reduce your intake of fat, you need even less because there is less fat being broken down. You will get plenty of vitamin E from all the vegetables and whole grains in your low-fat diet.

Vitamin pills don't prevent cancer. I've already told you about the study of smokers in Finland. Another study showed that Chinese peasants who took pills containing vitamins A and E and selenium had a 13 percent reduction in death rate from cancer.[23] Of course, that study was widely quoted to show that vitamin pills prevent cancer. They don't. You can't compare undernourished Chinese peasants with overfed Americans. The peasants in the study ate an extremely limited diet composed primarily of corn, wheat and pickled vegetables, which are very low in certain nutrients and high in cancer-causing molds that grow in stale foods. Americans eat a diet that has ample antioxidant vitamins and little mold. The National Cancer Institute did this study, and they do not recommend that Americans take vitamin or mineral supplements. They recommend eating a low-fat, high-fiber diet that includes lots of fruits and vegetables. There are many different phytochemicals in plants that have been shown to help prevent cancer, but scientists don't have the foggiest idea how to mix these chemicals into pills that will have the same effect as the food itself.

Extra iron may be bad for you. Do you remember the "tired blood" advertisements for iron pills? The Federal Trade Commission stopped them because the vast majority of people who are tired will not gain renewed vigor by taking iron. Popeye doesn't tell you this, but a diet rich in *iron and fat* can cause heart attacks. When you take in extra calories and fat, your liver manufactures large amounts of fat and cholesterol, which end up as the bad LDL cholesterol in your bloodstream. Iron and copper convert LDL cholesterol to oxidized LDL cholesterol, which forms plaques in arteries. A recent report from Finland showed that high iron levels can increase your chances of developing a heart attack.[24]

Doctors used to give iron supplements to people who were not anemic but had low blood levels of iron. They don't do that anymore. Less than 50 percent of the iron in your body is in your red blood cells. More than 50 percent of the iron is stored in your "iron reserves" — your liver, spleen, bone marrow and other tissues. You will not become anemic from iron deficiency until you have run out of all of your iron reserves. There is no evidence that iron deficiency harms you until you start to become anemic.

You can find out if you have high blood iron levels by asking your doctor to check blood iron, iron binding capacity and ferritin. Ferritin is the form of iron that is stored in your liver, spleen, bone marrow and other tissues. High ferritin levels usually mean that you have too much iron, but ferritin can be falsely elevated when you have arthritis or other diseases that cause swelling.

If you find that you have too much iron, you should eliminate any iron supplements you may be taking. The foods that are rich sources of animal fat — meat, chicken and eggs — are also rich sources of iron, and you will avoid these on a low-fat diet. You can also donate blood periodically.

Special Circumstances

You may need to supplement your low-fat diet with vitamin D, vitamin B$_{12}$, calcium or iron pills if:

- ◆ You are over sixty years old
- ◆ You are a strict vegetarian
- ◆ You are a woman at risk of osteoporosis

If you are over 60, you may need to take extra calcium and vitamins D and B_{12}. Researchers at Tufts University showed that most women over 60 lose calcium from their bones more rapidly during the winter months.[25] Vitamin D helps your body to absorb calcium from the intestines and also helps the bones to take up and hold that mineral. Most people get vitamin D by exposing their skin to sunlight. If you are over 60 and live in Boston, you probably don't get much sun in the winter, so you don't meet your needs for vitamin D and your bones grow thinner and weaker. Taking 500 international units of vitamin D and 1,500 mg of calcium helps to strengthen thin bones.

Another study showed that one in five people over 60 has atrophic gastritis, a condition in which the stomach does not produce much acid.[26] You need acid to absorb vitamin B_{12} from your food, and if you don't get enough B_{12}, your nerves will be damaged. If you're over 60 and itch or tingle or lack feeling in your arms and legs or can't remember things, ask your doctor to draw blood for a vitamin B_{12} test. If it's low, you should take large daily doses (1,000 mcg) of B_{12}. Plants contain no B_{12}.

If you are a strict vegetarian who does not eat eggs or dairy products, your diet lacks food sources of vitamin B_{12} and vitamin D and is probably too low in calcium. You should take supplements to cover these requirements.

If you are a woman at risk for osteoporosis, you may already be taking calcium supplements. Taking calcium pills can cause iron deficiency.[27] When calcium supplements are taken with meals, they markedly reduce the absorption of iron from the food. Have your doctor check your blood, and if you are anemic from iron deficiency, you should eat more fish or take iron pills. Take your calcium pills between meals and the iron pills with a meal.

Understanding Phytochemicals

Vitamins are not the only components of foods that help to keep you healthy. We have discovered hundreds of chemicals in plants (phytochemicals) that protect cells in your body and help to prevent cancer, and there are hundreds of thousands more whose functions have not yet been discovered. We have no idea how to combine all the beneficial chemicals into pills. That's why it is so important to eat a wide *variety* of fruits, vegetables, whole grains and beans, even if you choose to take vitamin supplements. A diet that is low in plant foods and high in vitamin pills is an unhealthy diet.

Fad Diets

Every year, another miraculous diet comes along, claiming to be the ultimate solution for losing weight painlessly. These diets make millions for their authors and leave dieters frustrated with yet another failed attempt to lose weight and keep it off. They usually promise that certain food combinations and chemical reactions will cause you to lose weight without effort. It would take a whole book to go through all the fad diets and the reasons why they don't work. Here are a few examples.

Low-carbohydrate or high-protein diets: The Atkins Diet, the Scarsdale Diet, the Doctor's Quick Weight Loss Diet and the Drinking Man's Diet were all based on restricting carbohydrates and eating mostly protein or fat. The theory is that your body will have to burn stored fat if it doesn't have any carbohydrates available. Your body prefers to burn carbohydrates during exercise, but severely restricting carbohydrates won't make you burn stored fat more than any other form of calorie restriction. It's more likely to leave you without the energy to exercise at all. The low-carbohydrate diets that tell you to eat lots of protein or fat give you far too many calories. All extra calories, regardless of their source, are converted to fat by your liver.

Cellulite diets: These diets are supposed to get rid of toxic wastes, which their authors claim cause the dimply fat deposits in your hips or thighs. They say that cellulite is a special kind of fat that won't respond to ordinary weight loss. That simply isn't true. The fat in the dimpled areas is the same as any other fat. Tiny ligaments run from your skin through the layer of fat to the muscles underneath. Extra fat pushes the skin up, while the ligaments hold the skin down. Small depressions form at the site of each ligament, causing the skin to look like the skin of an orange. The depressions will disappear when you lose weight.

Magical supplements: Lecithin, kelp, vitamin B_6, vinegar, fructose, whey — the list of supplements or special foods that are supposed to cause weight loss goes on and on. Anytime you hear that some nonprescription substance affects the way your body digests fat or alters your metabolism in some mystical way, be suspicious. While the Food and Drug Administration controls advertising claims and product labels, no one regulates the diet information that is spread through talk shows, newspaper and magazine articles and promotional pamphlets. Anyone can claim to be an expert with an amazing new diet miracle.

High-cost programs and gimmicks: The well-known commercial diet programs cost a lot of money and don't teach you to change your habits permanently. Their profits are higher if you keep coming back, buying their special foods and paying their monthly fees. Save your money; you'll do much better on a low-fat diet you can stick with forever.

Tony G. was one of eight dieters who reported their success with various programs in *Washingtonian* magazine (February 1992). After 12 weeks on their chosen program, here's how they stacked up:

Program	Weight Lost	Program Cost
Better Weigh (health club–based)	7 lbs.	$198
Zalman Nutrition Program (clinic)	10 lbs.	$895
Personal trainer	10 lbs.	$900 (my estimate)
Deal-a-Meal	15 lbs.	$95
Diet-to-Go (food delivery)	16 lbs.	$1,080
Jenny Craig	16 lbs.	$997
DietMate Personal Computer	25 lbs.	$395
Dr. Gabe Mirkin's Low-Fat Diet	**26 lbs.**	$0
Courtesy Washingtonian *magazine*		

Tony lost the most weight, using the diet he heard on my radio show, and it didn't cost him a penny. He said: "This diet has meant saying good-bye to Egg McMuffins, bacon double cheeseburgers, sausage biscuits, and Popeye's crispy chicken, but hello to pants I haven't been able to wear in years."[28]

CHAPTER 6

All You Ever Wanted to Know About Fats

I f you are confused by all the health claims about different kinds of fat, you're not alone. Advertisements, magazine articles and television shows distribute misinformation and half-truths about fatty foods. You won't prevent heart attacks by eating lots of extra corn oil for its unsaturated fat, fish oil for its omega-3 fat or olive oil for its monounsaturated fat. On a low-fat diet, you restrict all types of fats. This chapter will help you understand the different kinds of fats and how they affect your body.

Types of Fats

All foods contain a mixture of the three different types of fats: saturated, polyunsaturated and monounsaturated. There are no foods that contain only one type. All contain the three types of fat in varying proportions and are classified by their predominant type (Table 3).

If you look at Table 3 (page 44), you will notice that meat is classified as primarily saturated, but only 52 percent of its fat is saturated. Meat also has 37 percent monounsaturated fat and 2 percent polyunsaturated fat. Olive oil is classified as monounsaturated because it contains 81 percent monounsaturated fat, but it contains the other two types also.

Fats are classified by their chemical structure. If you want to learn the chemical differences between the various fats, read the box on pages 44–45. However, you don't need to know the chemistry to understand how fats affect your body and your risk of disease.

Table 3. Types of Fat in Foods

Food	% Saturated Fat	% Mono-unsaturated Fat	% Poly-unsaturated Fat	Fat Classification
Meat (avg.)	52	46	2	Saturated
Chicken	36	42	22	Monounsaturated
Fish (avg.)	50	40	10	Saturated
Eggs	38	53	9	Monounsaturated
Whole milk	61	36	3	Saturated
Butter	61	36	3	Saturated
Olive oil	12	81	7	Monounsaturated
Corn oil	11	31	58	Polyunsaturated
Almond oil	9	70	21	Monounsaturated

A Quick Fat-Chemistry Lesson

You do not need to know the chemical structure of fats to understand a low-fat diet. For those of you who want a technical explanation, here it is. Fats are classified by how much hydrogen they have in their basic structures. Fats are nothing more than a string of carbon atoms tied together.

$$-C-C-C-C-C-C-C-C-C-C-C-C-C-C- \ldots$$

Each carbon atom has 4 arms which can attach to other elements.

$$-C-$$

All of the arms must be attached to something else. Fats can have hydrogen elements attached to the carbons.

$$
\begin{array}{c}
H\ H\ H \\
-C-C-C- \\
H\ H\ H
\end{array}
$$

All carbons have 4 binding arms. All hydrogens have one binding arm. Some carbons do not have hydrogen attached to them. Then they have to bind to something else, so they bind twice to the next carbon. This is called a **double bond.**

$$
\begin{array}{c}
H\ \ \ \ \ \ H \\
-C-C=C-C- \\
H\ H\ H\ H
\end{array}
$$

Saturated Fats

Saturated fats are found in all food sources of fat, but they are found in *large* quantities in meat, eggs and the tropical oils, such as coconut, palm and palm kernel oils. When you take in more calories than you need, saturated fats raise blood cholesterol more than the other fats (or, for that matter, anything else in your diet). Anything that reduces your intake of saturated fats lowers blood cholesterol. However, if you replace saturated fat with other types of fat, you will lower your cholesterol only a little.

Polyunsaturated Fats

Polyunsaturated fats are also found in all sources of fat. Vegetable oils are particularly rich sources. *Substituting* polyunsaturated fats for saturated fats reduces your intake of saturated fats and lowers blood levels of both the bad LDL and the good HDL cholesterol a little. However, eating

---

Fats are classified by how many double bonds they have and where the double bonds are located. Fats that have no double bonds are called **saturated.**

```
    H H H H H H H
    | | | | | | |
   -C-C-C-C-C-C-C- ...
    | | | | | | |
    H H H H H H H
```

Those that have several double bonds are called **polyunsaturated.**

```
    H H              H
    | |              |
   -C-C-C=C-C=C-C-
    | | | | | | | |
    H H H H H H H H
```

Those that have a single double bond are called **monounsaturated.**

```
    H H H        H H H H
    | | |        | | | |
   -C-C-C-C=C-C-C-C-C-
    | | | | | | | | | |
    H H H H H H H H H H
```

All fat chains have a carbon end and an acidic end. Polyunsaturated fats are further classified into where they have the double bonds. Those that have the double bond three atoms away from the carbon at the non-acidic end of the chain of carbons are called **omega-3's.**

```
    H H        H H H
    | |        | | |
  H-C-C-C=C-C-C-C- .......
    | | | | | | |
    H H H H H H H
```

---

extra polyunsaturated fat will *raise* triglycerides, the fats that are made by your liver when you take in more calories than your body needs.

Taking *extra* polyunsaturated fat can harm you in other ways also. Large doses of polyunsaturated fat increase your chances of developing cancers of the uterus, breast, prostate, colon and gall bladder, as I explained in Chapter 4. They can suppress your immunity so you are at increased risk of developing infections, and they can cause gall stones.

People with arteriosclerosis often have low blood levels of the essential polyunsaturated fatty acids (linoleic acid and linolenic acid), but that does not mean that you should try to take in more polyunsaturated fat by eating margarine, vegetable oils or bakery products. You can meet all your needs for polyunsaturated fat just by eating plenty of fruits, vegetables, whole grains and beans, and perhaps occasionally eating small amounts of olives, soybeans, nuts or seeds. Vegetable oils contain only calorie-rich fat, and the extra calories will be converted to body fat and cholesterol by your liver. You should avoid margarine and bakery products because their polyunsaturated fats are often partially hydrogenated, which can raise cholesterol even more than saturated fat.

Monounsaturated Fats

Monounsaturated fats are also found in every source of fat in nature. Almonds and olives are particularly rich sources. As with polyunsaturated fats, *substituting* monounsaturated fats for saturated fats reduces your intake of saturated fats and can help to lower blood cholesterol a little bit. When you substitute polyunsaturated fats for saturated fats, you lower your good HDL as well as your bad LDL, but substituting monounsaturated fats for saturated fats lowers blood levels of the bad LDL cholesterol without also lowering the good HDL.

Olive oil distributors claim that consuming olive oil reduces blood pressure and blood sugar levels, but there is no evidence to support those claims. It is reasonable to *substitute* olive oil for butter, but I emphasize again: if you substitute air for butter or olive oil, you will reduce your intake of fat and saturated fat even more. You don't need to eat *extra* fat of any kind. **You get all the fats your body needs when you eat plenty of fruits, vegetables, whole grains and beans.**

Omega-3 Polyunsaturated Fats

Polyunsaturated fats are subclassified into omega-3's and omega-6's. Omega-3's are found mostly in fish oils and in some vegetable oils, such as olive oil, soybean oil and rapeseed oil. Omega-6's are found primarily in vegetable oils.

Omega-3's do not lower cholesterol unless you reduce your total intake of all fats.[29] They do help to prevent clotting, the last step that completely obstructs the flow of blood when you suffer a heart attack. If you have arteriosclerosis or have had a heart attack, you will probably want to have added protection against clotting. However, it's even more important to restrict fats in your diet so you can begin to reverse the plaques.

You can get the maximum anticlotting benefit by eating fish twice a week. People who eat fish twice a week have a reduced incidence of heart attacks, but those who eat fish more often than that do not have any further reduction in heart attacks. One baby aspirin every other day provides the same anticlotting benefit.

Tropical Oils

Palm, palm kernel and coconut oils are loaded with saturated fats. The manufacturers of these oils claim that the saturated fats in *their* products are different from the saturated fats in *animal* products. They cite studies that show that the principal saturated fat in tropical oils, palmitic acid, does not raise cholesterol. They are wrong. The data show that palmitic acid doesn't raise blood levels of cholesterol *only* when the subjects have low blood levels of cholesterol and are fed a very low cholesterol diet of fewer than 300 mg of cholesterol per day.[30] When people eat a normal American diet, which contains lots of cholesterol, palmitic acid raises blood levels of cholesterol significantly. The main sources of tropical oils are bakery products, such as cookies, crackers, breads and rolls, and prepared, canned and frozen foods, such as breaded fish and prepared vegetables.

Hydrogenated Oils (Trans Fats)

Public pressure forced bakery manufacturers to markedly reduce their use of the tropical oils. But other vegetable oils have a very short shelf life, so bakers add hydrogen ions to the polyunsaturated fats to form partially hydrogenated *trans fat* vegetable oils, which stay fresh much longer. These molecules have different effects on the body and are chemically different from polyunsaturated fats that occur in nature because the hydrogen ions line up in a different way.

The Department of Agriculture has shown that trans fats raise LDL cholesterol as much as saturated fats do. Worse than that, eating trans fats can lower blood levels of the good HDL cholesterol that helps to prevent heart attacks. That's one of the reasons I recommend that you avoid all bakery products except pita bread and other fat-free breads.

Artificial Fats

Fat makes food taste good by making it feel good. Fat molecules feel smooth to your tongue, and any molecule that has a smooth texture can fool your tongue into thinking that you are eating fat. Today we have three types of fat substitutes: those made from animal protein, those made from starch and those made from a sugar-and-fatty-acid molecule that cannot be absorbed. I'm sure chemists will develop others.

One type made from animal protein, called Simplesse, is manufactured from egg white and milk powder. It is used in many different products, such as ice cream and frozen yogurt.

The artificial fats made from starch are called polydextrose and maltdextrin. They appear to be safe and are found in drinks, desserts and various diet foods.

The third type is called Olestra and is made by combining sugars and fatty acids into a molecule that cannot be absorbed into the bloodstream. It has not yet been approved by the Food and Drug Administration.

Do fat substitutes help you lose weight or lower cholesterol? Probably not. We know that sugar substitutes don't help you lose weight,[31] and I believe that fat substitutes will not help you for the same reasons. The key to losing weight is feeling full with fewer calories. Since neither fat substitutes nor sugar substitutes fill you up, you will eat something else that contains calories. The only food component that fills you up without containing calories is fiber, and all the foods made with artificial fats that I've seen so far are low in fiber.

Most desserts and snack foods made with artificial fats have lots of calories and very little fiber. You may be fooled into thinking they are low-calorie foods because the portion sizes are ridiculously small. One popular brand of fat-free pastry claims that a serving contains only 100 calories. However, there are sixteen servings in the 4-inch-by-8-inch pastry, so each serving is the size of one of your fingers. It tastes so good that I bet you can't eat just one finger. A reasonably sized portion is 400 calories, and if you eat the whole cake, that's 1,600 calories. All the extra calories are converted by your liver to fat.

Salad dressings and mayonnaise made with artificial fats are fine because they encourage you to eat lots of vegetable and fruit salads. Look for "fat free" on the label so you get the varieties with zero grams of fat; many "low-fat" dressings still have several grams of fat per serving.

Triglycerides, Diglycerides and Monoglycerides

Just when you thought you finally understood all the different types of fats, along come these intimidating terms. Actually, these words just

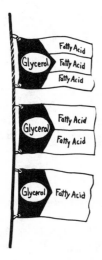

Fig. 4. Triglyceride means "three fats." Ninety-nine percent of the fats you eat are triglycerides.

describe the chemical structure of fats, and you do not need to be concerned about them.

Triglycerides are "three fats." They have a chemical structure shaped like an E formed by a straight vertical line and three horizontal lines, each comprising a fatty acid (Figure 4). Monoglycerides and diglycerides have the same single vertical line of the E, but monoglycerides have only one horizontal fatty acid and diglycerides have two.

All three glycerides affect your body in the same way. They all have 9 calories per gram and are broken down to form the same building blocks that are absorbed from your intestines into your bloodstream.

Almost all of the fat in foods is in the form of triglycerides. Monoglycerides and diglycerides together make up less than 1 percent of the fat you eat. They are added to bakery products to make them taste smooth, and to peanut butter to prevent the oil from separating out. They are added in such small amounts that they contribute an insignificant amount of fat to your diet. However, they are usually found in very high fat foods. Check the *total fat content* on the label.

Conclusions

What does all this information about fat mean to you? Don't be confused by the chemical terms or misled by people who want to sell you something. One simple principle should guide you: **restrict all kinds of fat.** If you want to lose weight or lower your cholesterol, you should limit your intake of all types of fat to no more than 20 grams per day.

CHAPTER 7

Food Facts and Fiction

Y ou can't prevent heart attacks by eating oat bran, walnuts, wine or anything else. You also can't cause a heart attack by eating butter, bacon, meat or pizza. No single food causes heart attacks or any other disease, and no single food prevents them. You won't be taken in by all the claims you read if you remember this basic concept: **Taking in excess fat and calories is harmful and reducing your intake of fat and calories is healthful.** Low-fat eating is healthful because you take in far fewer calories without feeling hungry. It's as simple as that.

Don't Waste Your Money

Why do we see so many newspaper and magazine articles about the special health benefits of one food or another? Usually it's because someone wants you to spend your money. As a member of the media, I constantly receive publicity packages from food producers associations and special interest groups, touting studies that support their particular product. These press releases get turned into articles by eager writers and editors who need to fill their pages. As a consumer, you need to remember that while laws control the claims that can be made in advertising, nobody regulates the content of news articles or radio and television reports. If it sounds too good to be true, it probably is.

Oat Bran Is Not a Medicine

A study in the *Journal of the American Medical Association* was widely quoted to show that oat bran prevents heart attacks. People with high cholesterol levels ate 1⅓ cups of oat bran each day, and their average cholesterol went from 223 to 218.[32] That's a lot of gas for a trivial drop in cholesterol.

Oat bran contains soluble fiber that binds to bile acids in the intestines and carries them from your body. Bile acids are used by your liver as building blocks to form cholesterol. You should eat lots of fiber, which is found in fruits, vegetables, beans and whole grains, including oats. Oat bran is a perfectly good source of fiber, but there's nothing magical about it. An oat bran muffin that contains 25 grams of fat will do far more harm than good.

Soybeans Won't Lower Cholesterol

Several reports claim that soybean products such as tofu lower cholesterol. They won't, unless you also reduce your intake of fat. Soybeans are low in saturated fat but high in polyunsaturated fat: 1 cup of cooked soybeans contains 10.3 grams of fat, compared to 0.6 grams in a cup of kidney beans. *Substituting* soybean products for meat or chicken can lower cholesterol a little,[33] but eating *extra* soybeans will raise it.

Nuts Do Not Prevent Heart Attacks

Several newspapers reported that an article in the *Archives of Internal Medicine* showed that eating nuts prevents heart attacks. The study showed no such thing.[34] Thirty-one thousand Seventh-Day Adventists were asked how often they ate certain foods. Those who reported that they ate nuts more than five times a week had fewer heart attacks.

All Seventh-Day Adventists are vegetarians, but some eat dairy products and eggs, while others do not. Whole-milk dairy products and eggs contain lots of saturated fat and cholesterol, two dietary components that increase blood cholesterol and susceptibility to heart attacks more than any other food components. Vegetarians who restrict dairy products and eggs have to get their protein from nuts and beans, both very low in saturated fat and cholesterol. Nuts do not prevent heart attacks, but restricting whole-milk dairy products and eggs does. It's no surprise that the publicity package on this study was distributed by a nut growers association.

Fructose Is No Bargain

Do you believe the claims that fructose will help you lose weight? Don't. Sugar in your bloodstream is called glucose, and it requires insulin to get inside your cells. Insulin causes your liver to make extra fat and your cells to store this extra fat. Entrepreneurs claim that fructose doesn't make you fat because it does not require insulin to get into cells. But to enter cells without insulin, fructose must be injected directly into your bloodstream. If you *eat* fructose, it ends up the same as granulated table sugar in your body. The fructose is converted to glucose in your intestines, or it is absorbed into your bloodstream and travels directly to your liver, where it is converted to glucose. It causes your pancreas to release insulin the same way table sugar does. Fructose also raises blood levels of triglycerides and uric acid higher than table sugar does.[35] Besides, it costs fourteen times as much as table sugar.

Granola Is Not Especially Healthful

Granola cereals have enjoyed an undeserved reputation for being a special health food. Of all breakfast cereals, they usually contain the most fat. In the 1850s, Dr. James Caleb Jackson created a cereal from broken bits of baked wheat and sold it under the name Granula. Dr. John Harvey Kellogg then made his own baked wheat cereal. He also called it Granula and claimed that it would cure many different diseases. When Jackson sued him for infringing on his patent, he reluctantly changed its name to Granola. Over the years, popular writers such as Gayelord Hauser and Adelle Davis revived the myth that granola cereals could be used to treat and prevent disease.[36]

Granola cereals are mixtures of processed grains, dried fruits, nuts, seeds and sweeteners. Claims of "all natural" and "no additives" are meaningless because all food is natural and the additives in breakfast cereals have not been shown to be harmful. The honey and raw or brown sugar in many granolas offer no health advantage over refined white sugar. Natural rolled oats taste like cardboard, so they are often fried in fat to make them taste better. Granolas may contain up to 40 percent fat, compared to almost zero for most breakfast cereals. Even the newer granolas labeled "low-fat" have more fat than many other cereals. If you want to eat granola, look for a box that says "nonfat."

Wine Does Not Improve Your Health

I receive huge publicity packets from the wine industry citing studies of the low heart attack rates among the wine-drinking French. They haven't persuaded me that wine prevents heart attacks, because wine is far from the only difference in our habits. For example, the French diet is much higher in antioxidant-rich fruits and vegetables.

If a person already has arteries partially closed with plaques, there is some evidence that wine may help to prevent clotting, the last step that blocks the flow of blood completely in a heart attack. There is no evidence that wine adds any benefits for people who use other anticlotting measures, such as taking a baby aspirin every other day or eating fish twice a week.

Studies from Japan isolated a chemical called resveratrol in red wine that helps to lower cholesterol in rats. There are no data to show that it lowers cholesterol in humans. Even if it is helpful, you don't need to drink wine to get it; you can drink purple grape juice.[37] Or better yet, you can eat whole grapes.

Ten percent of our population are potential alcoholics, so if they drink at all, they are likely to drink too much and suffer from cirrhosis, accidents, and breast and other cancers. Certainly you should not *start* drinking just because you think that it will prevent heart attacks. You shouldn't drink at all if you are trying to become pregnant or are pregnant, have a family history of alcoholism or breast cancer, take medications that are broken down by the liver, or work at a job that requires a high degree of alertness. Most people who do not fit into these categories can probably take up to two drinks a day without harming themselves. If you are trying to lose weight or lower your cholesterol, you need to remember that alcoholic beverages are high in calories, and all extra calories are converted to fat.

Don't Drink Juices, Eat the Fruits

Television infomercials and celebrity spokespersons extol the health benefits of vegetable juicers, claiming that juices cure cancer and a host of other problems. There is evidence that eating lots of fruits and vegetables may reduce your chances of developing cancer and heart attacks, but drinking juices is not more healthful than eating the whole fruit or vegetable. Most juicers remove fiber, so you lose one of the most important benefits of fruits and vegetables. Fiber helps to lower cholesterol and prevent gall bladder disease and constipation, and most people don't eat nearly enough. Juicing fruits and vegetables won't help you to lose weight either (see Figure 5). An 8-ounce glass of juice has 110 calories and no fiber, while a whole orange contains only 65 calories and has fiber to fill you up.

Fig. 5.

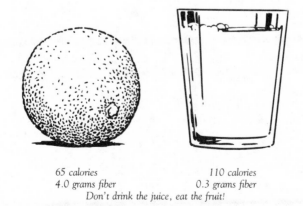

65 calories   110 calories
4.0 grams fiber   0.3 grams fiber
Don't drink the juice, eat the fruit!

Food Label Fibs

New rules issued by the Food and Drug Administration will make it a lot easier for us to separate truth from fiction in food labels and advertising. However, some foods, such as meats and dairy products, are not required to use the standard labels. Since manufacturers and advertisers want you to buy their products, I'm sure they will find lots of clever new ways to persuade you that their particular food is healthful.

Serving Size

The most common "fib" on food labels is the line that describes the serving size. If I buy a snack-size package of chips, I'm going to eat the whole thing. Yet the manufacturer apparently expects me to get two, four or even more servings out of one tiny bag. Table 4 shows you some of the serving sizes I found on packages of snack foods, and how they translate into grams of fat and calories in the whole package.

What Does "96 Percent Fat Free" Mean?

What do you think when you see milk, ice cream and yogurt that are called "96 percent fat free," or meat that is labeled "90 percent fat free"? They are high-fat foods, and if you are on a low-fat diet, *you shouldn't eat them.*

There are two ways to describe the fat content of food: percent by weight and percent by calories. Percent by weight should never be used. Even high-fat foods will have low fat percentages when you use that measure. All foods contain a lot of water, which has no calories, so the fat content is relatively *low* when you use percent by weight, even though it may be very *high* when you use percent by calories.

Table 4. Grams of Fat in Snack Foods

Item	Package Size	Serving Size	Grams of Fat per Serving	Calories per Serving	Total Grams of Fat	Total Calories
Potato chips	14 oz.	1 oz.	10g.	150	140	2100
Chocolate chip cookies	18 oz.	1 cookie	5g.	80	170	2720
Oreo cookies	20 oz.	1 cookie	2g.	50	108	2700
Tortilla chips	14.5 oz.	1 oz.	7g.	140	101.5	2030
Ritz crackers	16 oz.	5 crackers	4g.	80	112	2240
Cheese crackers	16 oz.	½ oz.	4g.	70	128	2240

A hamburger patty labeled "90 percent lean" (by weight) gets more than 50 percent of its calories from fat (see Figure 6). The United States Department of Agriculture recommends that "lean" beef contain no more than 23 percent fat by weight. That's 75 percent by calories, so "lean" beef is a very high fat food. Furthermore, only meat that is ground in federal or state packing plants must meet the USDA guidelines. Beef is usually ground in your local supermarket, which is not regulated. Most low-fat ground beef contains 10 percent fat by weight, which works out to more than 50 percent of the calories from fat. Forget the labels. There's no such thing as low-fat ground meat.

The same deception occurs when you buy ice cream labeled 96 percent fat free. The fat content is only 4 percent by weight, but it's 55 percent by calories. A single cup of 96 percent fat-free ice cream can contain 30 grams of fat.

"Light" Doesn't Mean "Fat Free"

Watch out for the label "light" on cheeses and other foods. The only cheeses you should include in your low-fat diet are made from skim milk. The label on one brand of mozzarella cheese reads "made from part-skim milk," yet it contains 12 grams of fat per ounce. Mozzarella cheese made from whole milk contains 13 grams per ounce. Only a few drops of skim milk need to be added to a quart of whole milk to make "part-skim" cheese.

The average cheese supplies 75 percent of its calories from fat. A low-fat cheese usually has 55 percent of its calories from fat. According to the new Food and Drug Administration guidelines, "fat free" means that the cheese has less than half a gram of fat per serving, "very low fat" means fewer than 4 grams of fat per serving, and "low fat" means that the product has one-third less fat than the regular product. Some manufac-

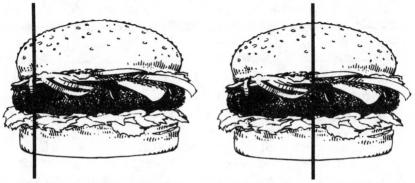

Fig. 6. Ground meat labeled "10% fat" by weight is 50% fat by calories. There is no "low-fat" hamburger.

turers remove the saturated animal fat in the cheese and then add primarily unsaturated vegetable fat back into the product. Even though these cheeses are free of cholesterol, they usually contain as much fat as the original product.

Chicken Is Not a Low-Fat Food

Creative advertising has led most Americans to believe that chicken is a low-fat food. It's not. Dark chicken contains the same amount of fat as beef, and the light meat isn't a whole lot better. Chicken has just as much cholesterol as beef, and neither has any fiber. Fried chicken has twice as much fat as beef.

One cup of dark chicken with the skin and fat removed contains 14 grams of fat, or three-quarters of the total fat allotment for one day for a person on a low-fat diet. One 8-ounce chicken breast with the skin and fat removed contains 6 grams of fat and 146 milligrams of cholesterol. You can eat chicken occasionally on a low-fat diet, but not an unlimited amount.

Two dietitians wrote a letter to the *New England Journal of Medicine* claiming that chicken contains the same amount of fat whether the skin is removed before or after cooking.[38] The *Nutrition Action Health Letter* found out that the figures were from an unpublished analysis of five chicken breasts by the National Broiler Council, an association of chicken producers.[39] That sounds to me like the foxes guarding the hen house. Even if the data are accurate, the story is really a subterfuge to hide the fact that chicken is not an especially heart-healthy food — no matter how you cook it.

Low-Cholesterol Eggs?

Some egg producers claim that *their* eggs are so low in cholesterol that you can eat a dozen a week without raising your blood cholesterol level. What they don't tell you is that after you eat the amount of cholesterol found in one egg, eating more will not raise your blood cholesterol further — as long as you don't increase your total calories. So their claim is true for *all* eggs.

As I explained in Chapter 5, your liver balances the amount of cholesterol in your bloodstream as long as you keep your total number of calories constant. When you eat more cholesterol, your liver makes less, and when you eat less cholesterol, your liver makes more. If you go from eating no cholesterol at all to eating the amount of cholesterol found in one egg (without changing your total calories), your blood cholesterol will go up a little. After that, no matter how much additional cholesterol you eat (again, without increasing total calories), you will not raise your blood cholesterol.

The cholesterol in eggs is not the problem. It's the fat. Those twelve eggs contain 72 grams of fat. When you take in extra fat, your liver manufactures extra cholesterol.

Low-Fat Milk

Whole milk contains 3.5 percent fat by weight. Since milk is mostly water, and water contains no calories, 3.5 percent of the weight equals 55 percent of the calories. A cup of whole milk has 8.5 grams of fat and 159 calories (see Table 5).

"Low-fat" milk has 2 percent fat and is still a high-fat food. Forty percent of its calories come from fat, and 1 cup contains 5 grams of fat and 145 calories. That's one quarter of your 20 grams for the whole day. The only milk that is truly low fat is *skim milk*. A cup of skim milk has 0.2 grams of fat and 88 calories.

The fat content of all dairy products is the same as that of the milk used to make them. Any dairy products you eat on a low-fat diet — including yogurt, cheese and cottage cheese — should be made from skim milk. Don't be deceived by "low-fat" labels on dairy products; the only ones you want are "no-fat."

"Low-Fat" Foods Can Defeat You

Food manufacturers know that many people are trying to cut down on fat, so they are producing lots of new "reduced-fat" or "fat free" versions of their high-fat foods. They're OK for occasional treats, but **you will defeat your low-fat diet if you eat a lot of these foods.** Manufacturers replace the fat with other sources of calories to make their products taste good. Low-fat cookies and pastries are usually loaded with sugar and egg whites, which are both dense sources of calories. Many of the low-fat versions

Table 5. Fat Content of Milk

Product	% Fat by Weight	% Fat by Calories	Grams of Fat in 1 Cup	Calories in 1 Cup
Whole milk	3.5%	55%	8.5	159
2% "low-fat" milk	2%	40%	5	145
Skim milk	0%	2%	.2	88

contain almost as many calories as the regular food. For example, Reduced Fat Oreo Cookies have 1.7 grams of fat and 47 calories a serving, while the regular Oreo has 2.3 grams of fat and 53 calories. The Hostess Light Twinkie contains 1.5 grams of fat and 120 calories, compared to 4 grams of fat and 140 calories in a standard Twinkie. Nabisco cuts the fat in their Fig Newtons from 1.3 grams in the regular cookie to 0 grams in the Fat-Free version, but both cookies contain 55 calories. These are all high-calorie foods and none of them contain significant amounts of fiber, so you will eat a lot without feeling full.

Food Claims We Haven't Heard Yet

The leadership of the Food and Drug Administration has taken strong action to limit deceptive claims and provide reliable information on food labels. However, food manufacturers want you to buy their products, and I'm sure they will think up ways to get around the new rules. You will be well armed against future misinformation if you focus on fruits, vegetables, whole grains and beans and avoid foods that contain more than 2 grams of fat per serving. In the next chapters I'll show you **how to make the food that's good for you taste so good** that you won't be led astray by clever advertising.

How to Make Low-Fat Food Taste Good

When I told **Rose P.** that she needed to go on a low-fat diet to control her diabetes, I thought she would die of a broken heart. Cooking was her life. She had spent many years running a catering service, and now that she was retired, her greatest joy was preparing fancy meals and desserts for her husband, children and grandchildren. We talked about some of the wonderful flavors of fresh vegetables, spices and herbs and came up with a lengthy list of her favorites. I challenged her to see if she could invent some new recipes using these low-fat ingredients. When she came back for her monthly checkup, she was all smiles. She had lost six pounds and got rave reviews from her family for her special new dishes. Best of all, they told her, "What we love most is having a healthy grandma."

My low-fat diet works where other diets fail because you don't ever need to feel hungry. Just as important, you can learn to make low-fat food taste delicious.

Most of my patients have a hard time imagining that they will ever enjoy the foods on my low-fat diet. Most of them like fruit but think vegetables are boring and seldom eat beans or whole grains. Like them, you probably learned to cook using a lot of fat, and most of your favorite prepared foods that you grab off the supermarket shelves are loaded with fat. When you switch to low-fat eating, you need to learn some new cooking techniques and change your shopping and meal-planning habits. This chapter explains my easy tricks for creating an endless variety of appetizing meals.

Flavor Full Principles

Low-fat meals can be as simple or as creative as you want them to be. Sometimes you need to put a meal together quickly, with a minimum of fuss. Other times you will feel like making something fancy or trying a new recipe. Whether you are preparing a quick lunch or a holiday meal, consider a few basic principles for making food taste good: variety, contrast, texture and visual appeal.

Variety

Foods taste better if you combine lots of flavors. Plain beans are dull. But beans cooked with onions and green peppers, seasoned with chili powder and served over brown rice are delicious! It's hard to go wrong when you combine different kinds of vegetables, grains and beans. The flavors complement each other, and the whole is tastier than the sum of the parts.

If you had to eat the same foods every day, you would soon rebel against your low-fat diet. Variety is important for good nutrition, too. If you eat lots of different fruits, vegetables, grains and beans over the course of a week, you can feel confident that you are getting all the nutrients, vitamins and minerals you need.

So many different combinations are possible that you never need to get bored. Don't be afraid to try unfamiliar fruits or vegetables, and take advantage of the fresh produce that's in season to vary your menus. If you find yourself in a rut, try preparing one of your favorite dishes with a completely different seasoning or spice.

I start my day by mixing three or four kinds of cereal in my bowl. Lots of my favorite recipes have long lists of ingredients because I like variety in every dish. Don't be intimidated; you just keep adding things to the pot, and it won't matter a lot if you leave something out or make substitutions. Soon you'll be creating your own recipes!

Contrast

We enjoy different combinations of food because the contrast keeps our senses alert. Just as your mouth becomes accustomed to something smooth, you introduce something crispy. Surprise! In the same way, our senses enjoy other contrasts — hot and cold, spicy and bland, sweet and sour. Your meals will be much more interesting if you plan for contrast.

One easy way to bring contrasting elements to your table is to use condiments. In many of the world's great cuisines, food is served with little dishes of condiments so each diner can customize his meal to his own taste. Mustard, catsup, pickles and hot sauces are standard condiments in the United States; look to your favorite ethnic restaurants for dozens of other ideas. You will see salsa on the table in a Mexican restaurant; hot pickles and cooling yogurt raitas in Indian restaurants; wasabi and pickled ginger served with Japanese dishes; kimchee with Korean food; fish sauce in a Vietnamese restaurant — the possibilities are almost endless.

Texture

Texture is another key to making low-fat food taste good. Fruits, vegetables, whole grains and beans have lots of different, interesting textures. Don't cook them to the point of mushiness or they will all feel the same.

Most vegetables taste best when they're crisp-tender. Check brown rice and other grains toward the end of their cooking time to make sure the grains are still separate and a little bit chewy. Then take them off the heat and remove the cover so they won't get too soft. Cook your pasta *al dente* — a little springy and firm to the bite.

If you serve a main dish with mostly soft ingredients, such as a soup or chili, complement it with a crisp green salad and crusty French bread, pita toasts or fat-free corn chips.

Visual Appeal

Food tastes better if it looks good. Your food doesn't have to look like a magazine photograph, but you can use some of the same techniques to stimulate your taste buds. Let the many bright colors in your produce department inspire artistic compositions for your table. If your main dishes don't have a lot of color contrast, add a bowl of bright fruits or vegetables, such as sliced red bell peppers, broccoli florets, berries or grapes. They'll liven up the table, and I bet they'll get eaten, too.

Take a little extra time to arrange food attractively on the plates, adding sprigs of fresh herbs, orange slices or raw vegetables as a garnish. A nice table setting, a few flowers and a little candlelight can turn a simple meal into an occasion.

Exploring Ethnic Cuisines

You can learn many lessons about variety, contrast, texture and visual appeal from ethnic restaurants and cookbooks. I always like to try new foods and experience new taste sensations. Your repertoire of low-fat dishes will be much more interesting if you are willing to venture into the cuisines of other countries.

Many inspiring ideas can be gleaned from the Asian, Indian and Hispanic diets that have been traditionally based on beans, grains and vegetables. Some Asian dishes are very low in fat, but Hispanic and Indian recipes usually need to be modified to eliminate the high-fat ingredients and cooking methods. You will still be able to capture the special flavors by using the traditional seasonings and some exotic ingredients.

Explore the ethnic food sections of your supermarket for unusual ingredients. Better yet, look for the specialized ethnic grocery stores that can be found in all large cities and many smaller communities. I love to browse through the aisles and buy a few items I've never tried before. Some of my experiments are more successful than others, but that's part of the fun. I've included some "exotic" recipes in Chapter 13 to get you started; look for the special symbol ▓ that denotes unusual ingredients.

Spices and Seasonings

When you take away fat, you need something else to make food taste good. Spices and seasonings are the secret of success! A well-stocked spice rack makes low-fat cooking exciting. You can vary the mild flavors of beans, grains and many vegetables in endless ways with spices, herbs and seasonings. Be adventurous!

I enjoy very spicy and peppery-hot foods. If you're timid about the amount of spice in some of my recipes, start out with a little bit, taste and add more until it seems just right to you. If you think you can't digest spicy food, try using just a fraction of the spices in one of my low-fat recipes and eat a very small quantity at first. You may find that your problem was with rich food, not the spices.

The next few pages list some of my favorite seasonings and spice blends, with ideas about how to use them. When you start to explore low-fat cooking, I know you'll find lots more.

Peppers

Black pepper is a wonderful flavor enhancer for salads, soups, vegetable stews and seafood dishes. If you don't already have one, invest in a good pepper grinder and a jar of peppercorns. Grind the pepper at the last minute before serving or at the table to enjoy its full flavor and fragrance.

Red pepper seasonings come in several forms — all hot. You can use dried pepper flakes, ground cayenne pepper, fresh or dried whole pepper pods or one of the hot pepper sauces such as Tabasco. Many of my recipes include red peppers. Add a little red pepper near the beginning of the cooking time, then check the "heat" after about ten minutes. You can always add more. If you get more heat than you like, dilute the dish with more of the cooking liquid or add some starchy vege-

If You Have Ulcers or Other Stomach Problems

I want you to be able to enjoy all of my favorite spicy recipes. If you think you can't digest spicy foods or any of the other foods on a low-fat diet, here's some important information that could change your life. **Eighty percent of ulcers and other common stomach problems can be cured with antibiotics.** If you have belching, burping, a sour taste in your mouth, or pain in your stomach that gets worse when you're hungry and better when you eat, you may have too much stomach acid. If you have these symptoms, your doctor should order an x-ray to help rule out a cancer and check for an ulcer, and you should get a blood test to see if you are infected with a bacterium called *Helicobacter pylori*. If the blood test shows infection, you can be cured by taking three drugs, metronidazole, amoxicillin and omeprazole, for one week. Repeat the blood test 12 weeks after you finish treatment. If the *Helicobacter* titre is still high, you may need a second course of antibiotics.

tables such as potatoes. If your mouth burns from too much hot pepper, try eating an orange.

Spice Blends

Spice mixtures are indispensable for quick, tasty low-fat cooking. You can buy good curry powder, chili powder and Cajun spices, or you can mix your own. I use prepared blends when I'm in a hurry and experiment with my own mixtures when I have time to make something special. You'll find these and many other spice blends in the spice section or the international foods section of your supermarket. Don't be afraid to try something new.

Chili powder is a blend of dried chiles, oregano and cumin and ranges from mild to hot. The mild ones usually have more flavor, and you can add heat with cayenne pepper to suit your own taste. Chili powder goes well with beans and is the basic seasoning for vegetarian chilies.

Curry powder has that wonderful fragrance you associate with Indian food. Indian cooks always mix their own spices, and you can, too, but packaged curry powder is a great shortcut for quick vegetable "curries." Try one of my basic vegetable curry recipes and then invent your own vegetable combinations, using whatever looks good in your produce department. Or add it to fat-free mayonnaise to make any bean or seafood salad special.

Five-spice powder is a Chinese blend of star anise, fennel, cloves, cinnamon and ginger. Sprinkle a little on fish before steaming or use it to season vegetables. You can buy five-spice powder in many grocery stores and in Asian markets.

Cajun spice mixes blend cayenne pepper, paprika, onion, garlic and various other spices into the secret weapon of Louisiana chefs. Several different blends are offered by major spice makers, labeled for use with vegetables, seafood or meat. Try a few until you find one you like. Use Cajun spices to create tasty vegetable stews and gumbos or to coat fish fillets before broiling to capture the taste of "blackened" fish.

Harissa (Moroccan spice) is one great spice mix you can't buy in the grocery store. It's a combination of cayenne pepper, cumin, fresh garlic and caraway seed. Commercial brands (when you can find them) are made with oil, so you'll need to make your own. One batch lasts a long time. My recipe is on page 307. Season mixed vegetables with harissa and serve them over couscous for an exotic treat.

Berbere is another hot spice blend that is African in origin, not quite as fiery as harissa. It includes several "sweet," fragrant spices such as cinnamon and allspice and is wonderful for seasoning vegetable stews. My version is on page 307.

Dried Herbs and Spices

In addition to the basic spice mixes and peppers, keep a variety of dried herbs and spices on hand. Buy spices and herbs as you need them for specific recipes, then experiment with new uses for the ones you like. You'll find dozens of kinds in your supermarket and even more in ethnic grocery stores. The ones I use most often are:

Allspice	Coriander	Oregano
Bay leaves	Cumin	Paprika
Caraway seed	Fennel seed	Rosemary
Celery seed	Ginger	Thyme
Cinnamon	Mustard	Turmeric
Cloves	Nutmeg	

Most dried herbs and spices keep a long time, but check them periodically for freshness. Your nose is the best test: if a spice lacks its distinctive fragrance, it won't add much flavor. Whole spices keep longer than ground ones, and you get a flavor bonus if you grind spices (like black pepper) fresh as you use them.

Fresh Herbs and Spices

Some of the most flavorful herbs must be used fresh. Dried versions may be available, but there's no comparison in the flavor. Dried basil and parsley flakes taste like dried grass.

Most supermarkets carry a good selection of fresh herbs, so you can buy them the week you plan to use them. If you have a home garden or a sunny windowsill, you can grow chives, basil and other herbs and snip them as you need them.

Basil. A natural partner for tomatoes, basil reminds me of licorice or anise. One of summer's great treats is vine-ripened tomatoes with a lavish amount of chopped basil. If you garden or have access to an Asian grocery store, try several different varieties of basil, including the ones with beautiful bright purple leaves.

Chives. This familiar member of the onion family can be snipped into salads, soups or any dish in which a mild onion flavor is desired. Garlic chives have broader leaves and a slightly stronger flavor.

Cilantro. Also known as Chinese parsley or fresh coriander, this fragrant herb is beloved in Hispanic, Asian and Indian cuisines. If you've

---

Grow Your Own Fresh Herbs

If you have a sunny windowsill, balcony or patio, you can grow herbs in containers. If you like to garden, add a special bed for herbs or mix them in a flower border.

The easiest way to start is with small potted plants purchased from your local garden center. Re-pot them in larger containers with drainage holes, set them in a sunny spot, keep them well watered and snip off leaves as you need them.

My favorites for easy growing and great flavor are basil, oregano, thyme, mint, chives and garlic chives. Parsley and cilantro are easy to grow but they go to seed quickly, so you need to keep replanting them.

Mint is nice to have on hand for cool summer drinks and salads. If you have an out-of-the-way place in your yard, even in the shade, you can start a patch of mint. Just don't put it in your herb garden or a flower bed — it spreads by underground roots and will crowd out everything else.

If you have space outdoors, put a few cayenne pepper plants among your herbs or tuck them in among flowers or shrubs. They are very pretty, and two or three plants will give you a year's supply of peppers. They can be used in chili and curry dishes or wherever you want a little added heat. If you live in a cold area, pull up the plants before your first frost, and let the peppers dry for use all winter.

---

eaten good salsa in a Mexican restaurant, you will recognize the flavor. Use it in chili, salads and Asian-inspired soups.

Dill. This feathery plant is as pretty as it is tasty. Use fresh sprigs in salads or snip it onto vegetables or fish before steaming. Steep dill sprigs in a bottle of vinegar and use it for salad dressings or for marinating vegetables.

Garlic. Please use only fresh garlic. Dried garlic and garlic salt don't taste anything like the real thing. Buy firm heads of garlic and store them as you do onions, in a cool, dry place. To peel a garlic clove, cut a small piece off each end, press the clove with the flat blade of your knife, then slip the skin off. Or use a good garlic press — no need to peel first. For a wonderful treat, try my roasted garlic on French bread (see page 313).

Ginger. Fresh ginger enhances steamed oriental vegetables or steamed fish, as well as curries and soups. Buy a small piece of root and peel the skin off a half inch of one end. You can then slice it, chop it into small dice or grate it on a fine grater. Gingerroot will keep for a few weeks in your refrigerator; it can also be frozen.

Lemon grass. Thai and Vietnamese cooks use lemon grass to flavor soups and cooking liquids. Look for it in Asian grocery stores. Don't bother with dried lemon grass; it's tasteless. To use fresh lemon grass, cut off the roots and slice pieces from the bottom 4 to 6 inches of the stalk. You may want to crush it before adding it to cooking liquid to get the maximum flavor. The rest of the stalk gets added to the stock pot or the compost heap — or just thrown out.

Oregano or marjoram. Fresh leaves of these herbs are much tastier than the dried ones. Add to tomato sauces, steamed vegetables or salads. Fresh oregano adds a special flair to my famous eggplant-tomato-bean casserole (recipe on page 136).

Parsley. Flat-leaved Italian parsley has more flavor than the curly kind. Use it to add flavor to soups and vegetable stews as well as for garnishing.

Rosemary. A very pretty and easy plant outdoors or in a pot, the narrow gray-green leaves of rosemary can be added to just about any vegetable dish.

Thyme. Especially good with green beans or zucchini. Add it to soups, stews and tomato sauces. If you grow your own, don't miss the special tang of lemon thyme or the beautiful silver-edged thyme.

Bottled Seasonings

Your arsenal of flavoring tools should include a variety of bottled sauces and seasonings. Almost all of the standard "wet" seasonings — such as mustard, Worcestershire sauce and horseradish — are fine on a low-fat diet. The only ones you need to avoid are those that contain oil. Check the labels.

Bottled seasonings can be used as cooking ingredients or added at the table. Look for unusual ones in the international section of the supermarket and in ethnic food stores. Experiment with inventive ways to use your old favorites and try some new ones.

A-1 sauce	Hoisin sauce
Catsup	Horseradish
Chili-garlic puree (Chinese)	Hot pepper sauces
Fat-free mayonnaise	Mustard
Fat-free salad dressings	Oyster sauce
Fish sauce (Thai or Vietnamese)	Soy sauce
Flavored vinegars	Worcestershire sauce

Adding Flavor with Cooking Liquids

As you'll see in the section on cooking techniques (pages 68–69), the basic low-fat cooking methods all use liquid: steaming, simmering and wet-sautéing. You can improve the taste of most dishes by using a flavored liquid rather than plain water.

Bouillon. I use bouillon cubes or granules constantly. The small amount of added flavor from a bouillon cube or two makes a big difference in the final product. Two chicken bouillon cubes go into the cooking water for brown rice, bulgur, couscous and almost any other grain. For soups or stews, use one cube for each 1 or 2 cups of liquid. Beef, fish or vegetable bouillon is fine, too. You won't need any additional salt. You can also use canned nonfat bouillon or consommé, but I find the cubes easiest to store and use.

Homemade stock. If you have the time and inclination to make your own soup stock, use it instead of bouillon cubes. My recipes for fish and vegetable stocks are on page 308.

Tomato sauce and juice. The tomato in its many forms is another powerful ally for the low-fat cook. Tomato-based liquids are indispensable in many soups, bean dishes and sauces. The flavor of tomatoes seems to blend other ingredients together, adding richness with zero grams of fat. My recipes use lots of tomato sauce, tomato juice and canned tomatoes with their liquid. Tomato paste, tomato puree or dried tomatoes work the same magic. If you have an abundance of fresh tomatoes in the summer, you can use them as a cooking liquid as well as in salads. Puree them in a food mill or cut the tomatoes in half and press them against a large-holed grater, then use the pulp and juice in your recipe.

Wine and beer. Wine is a classic cooking liquid that can add a special flavor to seafood or vegetable dishes. Beer is good for steaming shrimp or crabs. Include these beverages in your low-fat cooking repertoire only if having them in your kitchen doesn't create a temptation to overindulge. You'll defeat your low-fat diet if you use one can of beer to steam the shrimp and drink the rest of the six-pack yourself.

Citrus juice and vinegar. A little tartness in your cooking liquid can add just the right touch. We're used to vinegar and lemon juice in salad dressings, but the flavors are equally compatible with warm foods. Try adding a little lemon or lime juice to vegetable dishes near the end of the cooking time. One of my favorite black bean soups is made with orange juice.

Other cooking liquids. Bottled clam juice makes a good base for seafood soups and stews. Clam/tomato juice and vegetable juice cocktails can be used in place of plain tomato juice. You can also use the flavored liquids that are by-products of cooking, such as the water left over from soaking dried mushrooms or steaming vegetables. Instead of throwing away the shells when you peel shrimp, cook the shells for a few minutes in a cup or two of water. Then strain the liquid and add it to soup or measure it into the cooking water for brown rice.

Low-Fat Cooking Methods

Every recipe my mother taught me started with "Sauté a chopped onion in butter." When you switch to a low-fat diet, you'll need to rethink your cooking methods. Deep-frying is out. Sautéing in fat is out. Stir-frying in oil is out. Casseroles baked with fat-laden toppings are out.

That's the bad news. The good news is that if you can boil water, you can make **any** of my recipes. Most low-fat cooking uses three simple water-based cooking techniques:

Steaming. Food is cooked in steam that rises off boiling or simmering water. Steaming is good for vegetables that cook in a short time, such as asparagus. Put a small amount of water (a half inch or so) in a pot and bring it to a boil. Add the food to be steamed and cover the pot; reduce the heat and cook until the food is crisp-tender. Check occasionally to make sure all the liquid doesn't boil away. You can also use a special steaming pot that keeps the food out of the water completely, or an electric steamer — a great invention for the low-fat cook! I use mine constantly.

Simmering. Food is cooked gently in water or other liquid. Beans, rice and long-cooking vegetables are usually simmered. Generally, you start with enough liquid to cover the food, bring it to a boil and then reduce the heat to a gentle simmer. The pot may be covered or uncovered.

Wet-sautéing. Food is cooked quickly in a small amount of boiling liquid. Put ½ cup or so of liquid in the pot, bring it to a boil, add the vegetables and stir frequently. Add more liquid if needed to keep the food from sticking to the pot. Wet-sautéing is useful for softening onions, celery or green peppers before adding other ingredients. You can also "stir-fry" quick-cooking vegetables using the wet-sauté technique.

You'll also do a limited amount of **broiling, grilling, roasting** and **baking** — without fat, of course. Broiling or roasting vegetables such as peppers, onions, tomatoes, garlic and potatoes brings out entirely different flavors than you get from simmering or steaming. If you haven't tried roasted garlic yet, you're in for a treat. Consult the recipe section for specific instructions.

I'm particularly fond of broiled fish. When you broil without adding butter or other basting fats, check the food frequently so you don't overcook and dry it out. If you like, you can brush on a little lemon juice or fat-free salad dressing.

If you enjoy baking, the traditional recipes for French bread and sourdough bread are fat free. Angel food cake is also fat free, as is my recipe for banana bread (page 294). Keep these for occasional treats, though. Fresh-baked breads and cakes taste so good that it's hard not to eat the whole thing. These are low-fiber foods, so you can consume a huge number of calories without feeling full.

> **Richard D.** came to me after he had already seen several physicians and dietitians. He was taking niacin and lovastatin and was on what he thought was a low-fat diet, yet his total cholesterol was 250 with HDL 29 and LDL 155, and his triglycerides were 370. He was terrified because his father had died of a heart attack at age 43. He was in big trouble because an HDL of 29 would protect him against an LDL of only 90. I told him I suspected that he was eating too much food, since his triglyceride level was so high and because he packed 227 pounds into a 5 foot 7 inch frame. People on truly low-fat diets lose weight. Even though he had removed most of the fatty foods from his diet, he was eating tremendous amounts of fat-free pastries, yogurt, breads and pasta — as many as three bowls of pasta at a time. I taught him to eat as much as he wanted of the low-fat foods that are high in fiber, and to limit his intake of the low-fiber foods. Today his cholesterol level is 150 with an HDL of 25 and an LDL of 90. He is off medication, his triglycerides are under 200 and he weighs 165 pounds.

Bean Basics

Beans are the cornerstone of a low-fat diet. When you eliminate meat and most dairy products, as I recommend, beans will be your most important source of protein. If you are not already acquainted with the many varieties and uses of beans, my recipes will help you get started.

Every supermarket carries a wide array of dried beans and several kinds of canned beans. You can use them all in unlimited amounts except soybeans. One cup of cooked soybeans contains 10.3 grams of fat, while other beans have about 1 gram of fat per cup.

If you venture into ethnic food stores — especially Indian or Hispanic ones — or a health food store, you will find even more varieties. Bean flavors are similar enough that you can substitute one type for another in most recipes without fear of failure. You may have no idea how long a new kind of bean will take to cook, but the method is always the same (see below). Just check the beans periodically until they are tender.

Purists insist that dried beans are superior in taste and nutritional value, while convenience-minded cooks may never use anything but canned beans. I use both — constantly.

Canned beans are economical and versatile. My favorite canned varieties are kidney beans, black beans and chick peas, although I usually have a few cans of other types in stock as well. Chick peas go into salads (always), soups and vegetable stews. They are also good straight from the can or marinated in salad dressing for snacking or as an appetizer. Black beans and kidney beans make excellent quick chilis or salads.

If you're using canned beans in a salad, drain the liquid and rinse the beans. For most other uses, the bean liquid in the can goes right into the pot.

Dried beans just take a little planning ahead. Advantages of cooking your own are even greater economy — where else can you get 5 cups of high-quality protein for less than a dollar? — and the ability to cook them to just the stage of doneness you desire.

Dried beans cook best if you soak them before cooking. Cover them with water in a large pot and let them sit overnight. Drain off the soaking water and cook according to the instructions below.

To de-gas dried beans: If you're bothered by gas when you eat beans, try this simple cure for your problem. Put the beans in a large pot and cover them with water. Bring them to a boil and take them off the heat. This breaks the capsules surrounding the beans and allows stachyose, verbascose and raffinose, the gas-causing sugars, to escape into the water. Stir a couple of tablespoons of baking soda into the water and let the beans soak overnight. Drain the soaking water off the beans and rinse them several times. (If you eat the soaking liquid, you will cause unbelievable discomfort for yourself and those around you.)

Cooking: Dried beans can take a long time to cook. Count on an hour or two for most kinds. If the beans are very old, they can take a lot longer.

Cover the beans with plenty of water, bring to a boil, then reduce to a gentle simmer. After forty-five minutes or so, check frequently to see if they're tender and add more water if needed. Unlike most other vegetables, beans do not absorb much flavor from their cooking liquid. You can cook them in plain water and add them to a soup or stew when they are partially or fully cooked. If you are using the beans in a salad, drain them and let them cool.

Lentils and split peas cook quickly and do not need to be presoaked. They will be tender in about 20 minutes and soft enough to puree in less than an hour.

The ABC's of Whole-Grain Cooking

All grains are good sources of complex carbohydrates. Unfortunately, most pasta, breads and bakery products are made with refined wheat, which has had the nutritious germ and fiber-containing coating removed. You end up with lots of calories from foods that don't fill you up or have much nutritional value. The same is true of white rice: the fiber-rich bran coating has been polished away in the refining process.

There's nothing wrong with eating a cup of pasta or a few pieces of fat-free bread such as French bread or pita, but you can't eat unlimited amounts. That's why I recommend using whole grains. The fiber in whole grains will help you feel full and satisfied without contributing calories.

The whole grains I use frequently include brown rice, wild rice, kasha (buckwheat groats), barley, millet and bulgur. True grains are the seeds of grasses. When I talk about whole grains in this book, I include some foods that aren't technically grains but that we eat in the same way and that share the same nutritional qualities. For example, buckwheat is the fruit of a plant in the rhubarb family, not a grass. But it is very high in fiber and low in fat, and we prepare it and eat it like the true grains.

All of the common whole grains (and most of the uncommon ones) are cooked the same way. One cup of the dry grain is added to 2 or 3 cups of boiling liquid. The amount of liquid and the cooking time vary with each type of grain, as shown in Table 6 (page 72). You reduce the heat so the water simmers, cover the pot and let the grains cook without stirring. At the end of the cooking time, or when most of the water is absorbed, remove from the heat and stir with a fork to fluff the grains. Don't overcook! Whole grains taste best when they are a little chewy (like *al dente* pasta), not mushy.

An electric steamer or rice cooker makes cooking whole grains even easier. The pot never boils over or burns, and you can leave the house and come back to perfectly cooked grains. Follow the directions that

Table 6. Cooking Times for Grains

One Cup of Grain	Cups of Liquid	Cooking Time
Brown rice	2½ cups	40 minutes
Wild rice	3 cups	50–60 minutes
Kasha (buckwheat groats)	3 cups	15 minutes
Bulgur	2½ cups	20–25 minutes
Millet	2 cups	20 minutes
Oats	2 cups	5 minutes
Quinoa	2 cups	10–15 minutes
Barley	3 cups	30–40 minutes

come with your appliance for guidelines on the amounts of liquid and cooking times. If the manual doesn't cover all the whole grains you want to cook, use the instructions they give for brown rice or wild rice as a starting point.

Whole grains soak up the flavor of the liquid you cook them in. I *always* add some flavoring to the cooking water, even if it's just a bouillon cube (see pages 187–188). You can also add spices and herbs directly to the cooking liquid. Stir in a little turmeric or curry powder for a special flavor and a lovely golden color.

If you are making a soup or stew that includes whole grains, you can cook all of the ingredients together in the same pot to blend the flavors. Just remember that you will probably need to add some extra liquid to make up for the amount the grains absorb. You can use Table 6 as a guide for cooking times.

Getting Started on Your Low-Fat Lifestyle

W hen you decide to switch to low-fat eating, I recommend that you start right out eating fewer than 20 grams of fat a day. Don't try to cut back a little bit. Get the fat out of your kitchen and out of your life! Here are the six steps for switching to low-fat eating.

Step 1. **Learn how to count grams of fat.** It's easy. No percentages or complicated math. No record keeping.

Step 2. **Read through the list of all the low-fat, high-fiber foods you can enjoy.** Learn which foods are low-fat but also low-fiber, and which foods to avoid.

Step 3. **Map out a meal plan for a week.** Pick out a few new recipes to try.

Step 4. **Clean out your kitchen.** Get rid of temptation.

Step 5. **Shop low-fat.** Learn how to read a food label. Shop for your week's menus and stock up on low-fat cooking essentials. Buy lots of fruits, vegetables, grains and beans. Stay out of the meat and bakery departments and the "junk food" aisles.

Step 6. **Start your first day of low-fat eating.** You're on your way!

This chapter tells you all you need to know to follow these six important steps to your new lifestyle.

Counting Grams of Fat

Your goal on a low-fat diet is to eat fewer than 20 grams of fat each day. Every living cell is made with fat, so all the food you eat has fat in it. When a food label shows zero grams of fat, it really means less than 1 gram. Even a stalk of celery has a fraction of a gram of fat. You don't need to carry a calculator around with you. Here's my easy method of counting grams of fat.

The Basic 15 Grams

Don't bother to count the grams of fat in fruits, vegetables, whole grains and beans. Eat as much of these as you want to feel comfortably full and satisfied (except those few that are on the list of foods to avoid on page 79).

You can also have *five servings each day* from the list of low-fiber/low-fat foods (pages 76–78). You should have at least one serving of skim milk or yogurt each day, and a serving of seafood three to four times a week.

Count all these foods as your **basic 15** grams of fat per day.

5 Grams — Your Choice

Since you want to eat fewer than 20 grams of fat altogether, that means you have up to 5 grams more to use as you please. Anything else you eat that has 1 gram or more of fat on the label needs to be counted.

You don't have to use all 5 grams. You can have perfectly satisfying meals and snacks using just your basic 15 grams. But the 5 "choice" grams let you enjoy some of your personal favorite foods.

If you want to eat more than five servings of low-fiber/low-fat foods in a day, count each extra serving as 2 of your choice grams of fat. You can have that extra cup of pasta as long as you haven't used up your choice grams.

Foods for Low-Fat Eating

Instead of thinking about the foods you need to avoid, focus on all the wonderful foods you **do** eat on a low-fat diet. You eat lots of different **fruits, vegetables, whole grains and beans** whenever you are hungry. **Low-fat/ low-fiber foods** add variety to your meals, and you can learn how to use **seasonings and condiments** to make fat-free dishes taste delicious.

Fruits, Vegetables, Whole Grains and Beans

Most of the food you eat should be fruits, vegetables, whole grains and beans. These foods are loaded with fiber and water and are low in fat.

They are abundant sources of nutrients, vitamins and minerals. Beans have lots of protein as well.

You should eat a wide **variety** of fruits, vegetables, whole grains and beans each week so you will get the full range of vitamins and nutrients. If you eat lots of different **colors** of produce — red, orange, yellow and green — you'll get plenty of the important antioxidant vitamins A, C and E. Here's a list of just *some* of the vegetables, fruits, beans and whole grains you can choose from:

Vegetables

Artichokes	Fennel	Peas
Bean sprouts	Green beans	Peppers — all types
Beets	Green onions	Potatoes — red, white
Bok choy	Jicama	Radishes
Broccoli	Kale	Shallots
Brussels sprouts	Kohlrabi	Snow peas
Cabbage — green, red	Leeks	Spinach
Carrots	Lettuce — all types	Summer squashes
Cauliflower	Lima beans	Sweet potatoes
Celery	Mushrooms — all types	Swiss chard
Celery root	Mustard greens	Tomatillos
Chinese cabbage	Napa cabbage	Tomatoes — all types
Corn	Okra	Turnips
Cucumbers	Onions	Winter squashes
Eggplant	Parsnips	Zucchini

Fruits

Apples — all types	Grapes — all types	Peaches
Apricots	Guavas	Pears
Bananas	Kiwi fruit	Pineapples
Blackberries	Lemons	Plums
Blueberries	Limes	Pomegranates
Cantaloupe	Loganberries	Prunes
Cherries	Mangoes	Raisins
Cranberries	Melons — all types	Raspberries
Dates	Nectarines	Strawberries
Figs	Oranges	Tangerines
Gooseberries	Papayas	Watermelon
Grapefruit		

Beans

Black beans	Fava beans	Pinto beans
Black-eyed peas	Great northern beans	Red beans
Cannellini	Kidney beans	Split peas — green,
Chick peas	Lentils — brown, orange,	yellow
Cranberry beans	green	White beans
Dried lima beans	Mung beans	

Whole Grains

Amaranth	Bulgur	Quinoa
Barley	Millet	Wheat
Brown rice	Oatmeal	Wild rice
Buckwheat (kasha)		

A few kinds of vegetables, fruits and beans are high in fat. These are on the list of foods to **avoid:**

Avocados

Coconuts

Peanuts

Soybeans and soybean products, such as tofu or vegetarian "hamburger"

Low-Fiber/Low-Fat Foods

These foods add variety to your low-fat diet, but you can't eat them in unlimited quantities (see Table 7). Skim-milk products and some breads and sweets may have no fat, but they are also very low in fiber. They are dense sources of calories because they don't have much bulk (fiber and water), so you consume a lot of calories without feeling full. You can defeat your low-fat diet if you eat more than about five servings of these dense foods a day. Your body converts the excess calories to fat.

I encourage you to eat skim milk and fish because they supply some important nutrients. The other low-fat/low-fiber foods are not necessary, but they can be used in small amounts to add variety to your meals. Low-fiber/low-fat foods include:

Skim milk and skim-milk products (one serving = 1 cup). One serving per day is essential. Skim milk is an important source of protein, vitamins and minerals. I recommend a cup of skim milk with your breakfast cereal every day. Or have a cup of nonfat yogurt or cottage cheese. If you are a strict vegetarian and don't eat dairy products, you will need calcium and vitamin D supplements.

Table 7. Serving Sizes for Low-Fat/Low-Fiber Foods

One Serving =

1 cup skim milk
1 cup fat-free yogurt (about 100 calories of any skim-milk dairy product)
 	
4-oz. portion fish or shellfish
 	
½ cup pasta
½ cup couscous
1 fat-free pita bread
2 oz. fat-free French bread
   (about 100 calories of any fat-free, unsweetened, refined grain product)
 	
1 oz. gumdrops or jelly beans
1 12-oz. soft drink
½ cup fat-free ice cream, frozen yogurt or fruit ice
2 tablespoons jam, jelly or syrup
1-oz. piece fat-free pastry
   (about 100 calories of any sweet, fat-free food or alcoholic beverage)

Choose up to five servings of the low-fat/low-fiber foods each day as part of your basic 15 grams of fat. If you want more than five servings, count each extra serving as two of your 5 grams — your choice.
Be sure to include 1 serving of skim milk each day and 3 to 4 servings of seafood each week.

Seafood (one serving = 4 oz.). Eat three or four servings per week. Fish and shellfish provide protein, vitamins and minerals. Fish also contain omega-3 fatty acids that help to prevent clotting, the last step in a heart attack. Many kinds of seafood have fewer than 2 grams of fat per serving (see Table 8, page 78). However, you don't need to limit yourself to this list; choose whatever looks fresh and appetizing.

Refined grain products with 0 to 1 gram of fat per serving (one serving = about 100 calories). This group includes breads such as pita, bagels, French bread, English muffins; pasta, couscous and white rice.

These foods add variety to your diet, but you can't eat them in unlimited quantities. Figure a serving as about 100 calories. That's one medium-size pita bread or ½ cup of pasta or couscous. There's no excuse

Table 8. Low-Fat Seafood

Fish and Shellfish with 2 Grams of Fat or Less in Each 4-oz. Portion			
Clams	Halibut	Oysters	Shrimp
Cod	Lobster	Perch	Skate
Crab	Mahi mahi	Pollock	Sole
Croaker	Monkfish	Rockfish	Squid
Flounder	Mussels	Scallops	Tilefish
Grouper	Octopus	Sea bass	Whiting
Haddock	Orange roughy	Shark	

Fish that are high in fat include salmon, mackerel, herring, rainbow trout and pompano. Most of the higher-fat fish have darker flesh, while the white-fleshed fish are mostly low in fat.

for using white rice — brown rice tastes better and has fiber. I don't recommend the bakery products made with artificial fats because they are high-calorie foods that have very little fiber. The serving sizes are ridiculously small — a 100-calorie portion is usually about the size of your finger.

Sugar and sugary foods (one serving = about 100 calories). These foods include jams and jellies; fat-free candies such as jelly beans, gum drops or licorice; fat-free ice cream, sherbet, fruit ice, and frozen yogurt; soft drinks and alcoholic beverages. These are fine as occasional treats — in small quantities. Sweet-tasting foods add variety to your low-fat diet, but they usually have lots of calories and little or no nutritional value. A 100-calorie serving is 2 tablespoons of jam or 1 ounce of jelly beans.

Seasonings, condiments and "freebies." These foods are used in small quantities and have no particular nutritional value, but they help make your low-fat food taste good. Use your favorites as often as you like and experiment with new seasonings. Check the labels of sauces and condiments to be sure they don't contain oil.

Bouillon cubes or
    granules
Coffee
Diet soda
Fat-free mayonnaise
Fat-free salad dressings

Herbs
Horseradish
Hot pepper sauce
Ketchup
Mustard
Other bottled seasoning
    sauces

Pickles and relishes
Soy sauce
Spices
Tea

High-Fat Foods to Avoid

I consider any food with more than 2 grams of fat per serving *high-fat*. In addition to the foods on this list, be aware that most prepared "convenience" foods — whether frozen, canned or boxed — are high-fat. Also notice that the "serving sizes" on many high-fat foods are deceptively small. Check the label before you buy. Avoid:

All bakery products except no-fat breads

All dairy products except skim milk and fat-free yogurt or cheeses

All meats (yes, that includes chicken and turkey)

Avocados

Cookies, crackers and chips

Eggs

Mayonnaise and salad dressings (except fat free)

Nuts, peanuts and coconuts

Oils, margarine, butter, shortening and lard

Seeds

Soybeans and soybean products such as tofu

How to Plan Your Low-Fat Meals

Low-fat eating is easy if you learn a few basic meal patterns that you can assemble quickly without a lot of thought. You can then experiment with new recipes and original creations whenever you have time and inspiration.

Breakfast

I eat the same breakfast every day: cereal, skim milk and fruit. My favorite winter breakfast is oatmeal with raisins, super easy to make in a microwave oven. My cupboard contains lots of different kinds of cereal — all with 0–1 gram of fat per serving. Read the fat content on the label. The brands made with whole grains and lots of fiber are best. Add raisins or other fruit if you like. Beware of the granolas; they are loaded with fat. Even the ones that are labeled "low-fat" have more fat than you need in a breakfast cereal — 2 grams or more in a tiny ½ cup serving.

You can add variety to your breakfasts with no-fat breads or yogurt as long as you count your servings of low-fat/low-fiber foods. Bagels have no fat, but an ounce of cream cheese would add 10 grams. You can have waffles or pancakes made without butter, whole milk or eggs, but use a little syrup or fruit instead of butter. Most of the other traditional breakfast favorites are full of fat. Two eggs contain 12 grams of fat, 2 slices of bacon have 5 grams, ½ cup of hash brown potatoes has 11 grams, and a tablespoon of butter contains 11 grams. Start your day with cereal instead!

Lunch

Whether you eat at work or at home, lunchtime is a short break in your daily routine. I like to keep it simple. My favorite lunch is a baked potato with salsa or frozen mixed vegetables and tomato sauce warmed in a microwave oven. Leftovers of last night's soup, casserole or salad make good lunches, too. Or choose two or three items from the list below:

Fat-free canned or instant soup

Fruit salad

Green salad or raw vegetables

Nonfat yogurt

Orange, apple or any fresh fruit

Pita bread

Tuna fish (water-pack) with no-fat mayonnaise (optional): count as one of your 3–4 servings of fish per week

If you're used to eating in a cafeteria or restaurant, I strongly recommend that you switch to bringing your lunch from home. It's very hard to control what you eat when a stranger prepares your food. The section on restaurants on page 87 will help you manage an occasional lunch out, but you have a much better chance of success if you "do it yourself."

Dinner

Dinner can be as simple or as fancy as you like. I like to combine vegetables, grains and beans in a casserole or soup and serve it with a salad. In warm weather, my whole-meal salads are tasty and quick to prepare.

I usually make a big pot of one of my favorite recipes on the weekend. We eat it on Sunday and one or two nights during the week, and freeze the rest in individual meal-size containers. If you do this for a few months, you will stock your freezer with tasty low-fat food that's as easy to serve as those expensive, high-fat prepared foods from the supermarket. My recipes that freeze well are marked ▓.

A week of dinner menus. Use the week of sample menus below for ideas. Recipes for the starred dishes are in Chapter 13. The seven vegetable stew, curry, crab soup and my famous bean-eggplant-tomato casserole can be made in large quantities and frozen.

The chili, clam sauce with whole grains and Cajun fish fillets can be prepared in less than half an hour. The recipe section will help you plan lots of meals that you can fix in a short time. Look for the◐ symbol.

Monday

My Famous Bean-Eggplant-Tomato
   Casserole*
Super-Easy Coleslaw
No-fat pita bread
Five-Fruit Curry*

Wednesday

Clam Sauce with Whole Grains*
French bread
Tossed salad with no-fat dressing
Hawaiian Smoothie*

Friday

Couscous with Seven Vegetables*
Ginger-Pear Frappe*

Sunday

Lentil Curry*
Brown Rice*
Ginger-Steamed Vegetables*
No-fat pita bread
Easy Banana-Strawberry Sorbet*

Tuesday

Quick Chili*
Brown Rice*
Toasted Tortilla Strips* or fat-free
   tortilla chips
Fresh Salsa* (or bottled)
Shredded lettuce
Sliced oranges

Thursday

Cajun Fish Fillets*
Steamed asparagus
Wild Rice*
Grapes

Saturday

Crab Soup*
Romaine, mushroom and red
   pepper salad
French Bread with Roasted Garlic*
Banana Bread*

Snacks

You can nibble on fruit or fresh vegetables at any time of day. If you want more substantial snacks, you may prefer to eat several small "meals" throughout the day instead of the traditional breakfast, lunch and dinner. Read on.

Gorge or Graze?

Many people skip breakfast, eat a light lunch and then gorge on a large amount of food in the evening. This will cause cholesterol and weight to rise higher than a more reasonable eating pattern that distributes your food throughout the day.

Eating a single high-calorie meal is more fattening than nibbling the same amount of food in several small meals. That's because eating raises your temperature for up to four hours, so you burn more calories. If you eat once a day, you increase your metabolism for only four hours altogether. On the other hand, if you spread the same amount of food out over several small meals, you increase your metabolism all day long, so more calories are converted to energy and fewer to fat.

Exercising after eating increases your metabolism even more. An evening meal followed by television is more fattening than a morning meal of the same size that is followed by activity.

The 19 Meals for Dr. Gabe Rule

Here's the good news. If you follow your low-fat eating plan faithfully for 19 out of your 21 meals in a week, you can eat out once or twice and have anything you want. Be reasonable — don't stuff yourself — but enjoy your food without guilt. People who haven't been able to stick to diets in the past will find that this simple rule makes a big difference.

- You can eat at friends' homes without asking them to cater to your special food needs
- You can deal with a craving for a favorite food
- You can enjoy a lunchtime or evening at a restaurant with family or coworkers

Notice that I said eat *out* once or twice. Don't bring the ingredients into your house! When you order a bacon, lettuce and tomato sandwich at a deli, you eat two slices of bacon. If you make it yourself, you need to buy the whole package. Who's going to eat the rest of it? Two slices of bacon have 5 grams of fat; bring the pound of bacon into your home and you (or your spouse) will eat 65 grams of fat.

Cleaning Out Your Kitchen

This step will be hard for people who hate to throw things away, but you'll be doing yourself a big favor. Get a box or a trash bag and go through your refrigerator. Throw out the eggs, mayonnaise, salad dressings, butter, cheese and other dairy products except skim milk and nonfat yogurt. Get rid of any luncheon meats, bacon or sausage. Empty the ice cream, vegetables frozen in sauces and packaged frozen foods with more than 3 grams of fat per serving out of your freezer.

Then tackle your cupboards. Throw out bottles of oil, cookies, crackers, chips, nuts and other fatty snack foods, bread and pastry. Read the labels of your canned and packaged convenience foods, and get rid of any that have more than 3 grams of fat per serving.

You may want to donate your nonperishable items to a food bank or other charitable group. Or give everything to a neighbor with teenagers. However you do it, get them out of your kitchen.

Then make a commitment to yourself that you will not bring any more high-fat foods into your house. No oil, no butter, no meat or cheese, no eggs, no nuts, chips or cookies, no pastries. If they're not there, you won't eat them.

Low-Fat Shopping

Make a mental map of your favorite supermarket. You'll spend most of your time in the produce department, with trips to the seafood counter and brief stops in the bread and dairy sections. You'll also shop for whole grains, beans, canned and frozen vegetables, spices and condiments.

Learn to avoid whole sections of the store. Stay away from the meat department. Stay out of the aisle with cookies, crackers and greasy snack foods. Find out where the low-fat breads are kept in the bakery department and turn your back on everything else. Ditto the dairy department — you're only interested in skim milk and nonfat yogurt; there is no need to even look at the rest. Most prepared foods — TV dinners, frozen pizza, packaged casserole mixes, dessert mixes, etc. — are loaded with fat. Avoid those aisles altogether. Don't bother with the frozen diet entrees; they're expensive and the portions are so small, you'll still be hungry. You'll be filling your freezer with "fast food" you make yourself (see page 133).

Reading Food Labels

Train your eye to look for one line on the food label: **TOTAL FAT**. Most of the fat in your diet should come from your major sources of protein — beans and seafood. On all other items, if it doesn't say 0 grams of fat (or less than 1 gram), look for an alternative (Figure 7, page 84).

When you switch to low-fat eating, it's worthwhile to spend some time comparing brands. For example, some kinds of pita bread have as much as 3 grams of fat per piece, while others have 0 grams. Those 3 grams can make a big difference when you're trying to stay under 20 grams of fat per day.

It's also important to check the serving size. Some food manufacturers use portions that are ridiculously small to deceive you into thinking their food is low-fat or low-calorie.

You can ignore all of the rest of the information on the food label. I find the percentage values especially confusing, and I majored in math in college. There's no way to tell from the percentages whether the gov-

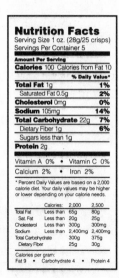

Nutrition Facts
Serving Size 1 oz. (28g/25 crisps)
Servings Per Container 5

Amount Per Serving

Calories 100 Calories from Fat 10

	% Daily Value*
Total Fat 1g	**1%**
Saturated Fat 0.5g	**2%**
Cholesterol 0mg	**0%**
Sodium 105mg	**14%**
Total Carbohydrate 22g	**7%**
Dietary Fiber 1g	**6%**
Sugars less than 1g	
Protein 2g	

Vitamin A 0%	•	Vitamin C 0%
Calcium 2%	•	Iron 2%

* Percent Daily Values are based on a 2,000 calorie diet. Your daily values may be higher or lower depending on your calorie needs.

	Calories:	2,000	2,500
Total Fat	Less than	65g	80g
Sat. Fat	Less than	20g	25g
Cholesterol	Less than	300g	300mg
Sodium	Less than	2,400mg	2,400mg
Total Carbohydrate		300g	375g
Dietary Fiber		25g	30g

Calories per gram:
Fat 9 • Carbohydrate 4 • Protein 4

Fig. 7. Food Label Reading Made Easy:

◆ *Look first at Total Fat. Is it under 3 grams per serving?*
◆ *Check Serving Size. Is it reasonable for you? You can ignore everything else.*

***Don't** use the % of Daily Value shown for fat; it's based on getting 30 percent of your calories from fat (more than 60 grams), and that's way too much.*

ernment thinks you should get more of that component — like vitamins — or less of it — like fat or sodium. When it comes to fat, the percentages on food labels don't apply to you at all because they are based on getting 30 percent of your total calories from fat. That's way too high. Keep your eye on the total grams of fat per serving and the serving size. You'll have all the information you need.

Stocking Up

After you've cleaned out your kitchen, restock your shelves with the staples of your low-fat meals:

In Your Cupboards

Canned and dried
vegetables and fruits
Canned beans
Canned tuna fish
(water-pack)

Cereals
Dried grains and beans
Juices
Nonfat salad dressings
and mayonnaise

Spices, seasonings and
condiments
Sugar, syrup, jam and
jelly

In Your Freezer

Frozen vegetables, fruits
and juices
Fat-free breads

. . . and a supply of your
own casseroles and
soups

Long-keeping vegetables	Carrots	Onions
and fruits, such as:	Celery	Oranges
Apples	Garlic	Peppers
Cabbage	Grapefruit	Potatoes

Make a List

The first few weeks, make a list of the ingredients you will need for the meals you've planned. Keep your kitchen well stocked so you can improvise when you wish. Buy lots of fresh fruit and salad vegetables each week. After a while, you will find that low-fat shopping is easy and you'll need to keep a list only for special items.

You'll be delighted to find that the ingredients of a low-fat diet are among the lower-cost items in the grocery store. Beans and whole grains are nutritional bargains. You are likely to find that the cost of a full basket of groceries is much lower than it was when you were buying meats, high-fat dairy and bakery products and lots of prepared foods. Use your savings to indulge yourself in the produce and seafood departments. Buy exotic or out-of-season fruits and vegetables, and treat yourself to high-priced lobster or crab once in a while.

Sources of Special Foods

You can get everything you need for low-fat eating at your supermarket. For variety, I encourage you to explore some other stores that have interesting low-fat ingredients.

Ethnic grocery stores. Get to know the Asian, Hispanic, Indian and other ethnic stores in your area. Many of them carry unusual fresh produce, dried beans, spices and other exotic ingredients. You may not be able to read the labels or communicate with the staff, but it's fun to take an occasional gamble. Here are some of the foods I look for in my favorite ethnic grocery stores:

- ◆ **Chinese:** Black bean sauce, bamboo shoots, bean sprouts, leafy green vegetables, long green beans, dried mushrooms, hoisin sauce, oyster sauce
- ◆ **Hispanic:** Beans, peppers, spices
- ◆ **Indian:** Beans, spices, pickles
- ◆ **Japanese:** Buckwheat noodles, dashi (fish stock), dried mushrooms, dried seaweed, canned tiny cocktail shrimp, wasabi (dried green horseradish), rice vinegar

- ◆ **Korean:** Kimchee (spicy pickled cabbage), red peppers
- ◆ **Vietnamese:** Noodles, fish sauce, fresh vegetables, peppers, cilantro, tamarind, basil (different varieties), fresh lemon grass, lime leaves

Produce stands and farmers markets. Fresh, locally grown produce is a special treat. Some tasty varieties of fruits and vegetables are available only at these outlets because they don't ship well. There's just no substitute for vine-ripened tomatoes or freshly picked sweet corn.

Health food stores. These can be excellent sources for unusual whole grains and beans. They are often sold in bulk at very reasonable prices. Just don't be taken in by claims of superior nutrition from organically grown foods or special supplements. And remember to read all labels for fat content. Many prepared vegetarian foods are very high in fat.

Challenging Situations

When you're on a low-fat diet, you need to be able to deal with some roadblocks that make it hard to follow your new eating patterns. Here are some suggestions for handling holidays, restaurants, airline food, and family members who don't share your eating habits.

Feeding a Family

Low-fat eating is easiest when everyone in your household is interested in a healthy diet. But if you have growing children or an unwilling mate, you will need to keep some high-fat foods in the house. Prepare the same low-fat breakfast and dinner for everyone and let them add higher-fat items at the table — butter, cheese, ice cream. They can eat whatever they want for lunch at school or work.

Try to buy foods for them that you don't like and won't be as tempted to eat. If your weakness is chocolate ice cream, buy them strawberry. Keep a cupboard and a refrigerator drawer of "their" food and stay out of it. It will take more will power, but you can do it.

A word for the unwilling mate: Even if you don't have a weight or cholesterol problem, your support can mean the difference between success and failure for your spouse. It's possible for him or her to avoid the fatty foods you insist on having in the house, but it can be very hard. Try my low-fat diet, at least for breakfast and dinner; you are likely to find that you feel better, too. If you care about your spouse's health, you will keep your house as a fat-free sanctuary and indulge your appetite for fatty foods when you are out of sight.

Restaurants

Virginia J. brought her husband, Fred, to see me because he weighed 240 pounds, too much for his 5 foot 8 inch height. I taught them about my low-fat diet and they appeared to grasp the concepts readily. When they returned six weeks later, Fred had lost only 2 pounds. Virginia had done a good job of removing fat from the household, but Fred was going out to lunch every day with his associates. It's OK to eat out occasionally, but five high-fat meals is too many. I persuaded Fred to take a low-fat lunch to work, and three months later, he was down to 215 pounds and on his way.

For that occasional meal out, remember the 19 Meals for Dr. Gabe rule. Once or twice a week you can eat whatever you like, as long as you follow your low-fat eating plan for the other 19 meals.

If your work requires you to travel or entertain a lot, you need to learn how to get a low-fat meal in a restaurant. Most restaurants are used to customers on diets and will try to cooperate. Find a restaurant with a good salad bar, and load up on fresh vegetables. Avoid the mayonnaise-based salads, cheeses, croutons, dressings and other high-fat items. If you're a regular customer, ask the waiter to keep no-fat (not low-fat) dressing on hand for you. A friend of mine carries a bottle of his favorite dressing in his briefcase.

Have some bread, breadsticks or a roll or two as long as you don't use butter. Order broiled fish for your entree. Ask to have it prepared with lemon juice instead of butter. Have steamed vegetables as an accompaniment, without added butter, and fresh fruit or fruit ice for dessert. Don't fall for the waiter's suggestion to bring "sauce on the side." If it comes to your table, you'll probably eat it. Have him leave it in the kitchen instead.

Airline Travel

Airline food is high in fat and not very appealing. One airline recently offered me a choice between an omelet with sausage and their "healthy breakfast." The breakfast included a package of granola, 2 percent low-fat milk, Touch of Butter spread, orange juice and an unlabeled muffin. The container of granola said "low-fat" in big letters, with 2 grams of fat per serving. I was outraged when I read that the tiny container had two servings! I guess I was supposed to pour half of it into my pocket and save it for the next day. Calling 2 percent milk low-fat is deceptive; whole milk has only 3 percent fat. The ½-cup carton had 3 grams of fat. The spread label announced that it was cholesterol free, but since it was all fat, the tiny packet added another 5 grams. The muffin, its top glistening with fat, probably had at least 10 grams. That's a total of 22 grams of fat, 2 more than I usually eat in a whole day.

You can use the 19 Meals for Dr. Gabe rule when you fly, but there's a much better solution. All airlines will provide meals to meet special diet needs, including low-fat meals, if you call ahead. If you travel a lot, tell your travel agent to ask for a cold seafood or fruit platter. You'll be the envy of your seatmates.

Even those little packages of nuts have 7 grams of fat. If it's a short flight, take along your own low-fat snack and pass up the peanuts.

Holidays

You can always use the 19 Meals for Dr. Gabe rule for a single holiday dinner. But in many families, holidays involve several days of large meals, coupled with frequent parties and gift foods. You can make the holiday foods you serve delicious, festive *and* low-fat.

Instead of laying out high-fat cheeses and crackers, try low-fat pretzels, toasted pita wedges and raw vegetables. Lobster, scallops, crabs and shrimp are treats that have far less fat than roast turkey, beef or ham. Garnish your foods with fruits, such as grapes, spiced apple rings, pineapple, lemon juice and orange slices; or use sweetened vegetables, such as carrots with honey or sweet potatoes with brown sugar. Serve lots of interesting salads with no-fat dressings. Skip the usual high-fat desserts and serve fruits, such as baked apples, pineapple glazed with brown sugar or a compote of oranges, grapes and apple slices.

If you have traditional family recipes that are important to your celebrations, see if you can adapt them to omit the fatty ingredients. Try some of the suggestions on page 89 for adapting your favorite recipes.

Start Cooking!

You don't have to be a great cook to make low-fat food taste good. Pick out a few of the recipes in Chapter 13 and try your hand. They're all easy and delicious. Once you get used to the idea of cooking without fat or fatty ingredients, you will be able to create lots of tasty dishes of your own. The possibilities are endless!

Adapting Recipes

Every family has its own special recipes. When you go on a low-fat diet, you may have to abandon some of your favorites, but others can be adapted to your new way of eating. Look over your recipes and pick out a few that have at least some of the ingredients of your new lifestyle — fruits, grains, vegetables or beans. Then try them using these tips for turning your regular recipes into low-fat gems.

- ◆ Eliminate the most common high-fat ingredients — oil, butter or margarine and eggs. You can substitute something else to add moisture if needed. Applesauce or mashed ripe bananas work well in some recipes for baked goods. A little stock, lemon juice or tomato juice makes a good substitute for the oil in vegetable or fish dishes.
- ◆ To replace nuts, try dried fruits such as apricots, dates or raisins, or a crunchy cereal such as Grape Nuts.
- ◆ For sauces, casseroles or soups that call for ground meat, try substituting cooked lentils or chick peas, or a chewy-textured grain such as kasha (buckwheat groats) or wild rice.
- ◆ Use yogurt cheese (page 313) as a substitute for high-fat cheeses or sour cream.
- ◆ Try fat-free salad dressings as a cooking ingredient in place of butter or oil. I'm still experimenting with these and have had some good results.
- ◆ If a favorite recipe calls for frying or sautéing, try steaming the same ingredients in a little stock or other flavored cooking liquid (see page 69).
- ◆ You may want to increase the amount of spices in your recipe, or if it seems bland without its fatty ingredients, you can try adding some new spices or seasonings.

How to Exercise

Bob R. had triple bypass surgery shortly after he retired. I warned him that surgery is a short-term fix and that if he didn't change his diet and get some exercise, he would soon have another heart attack. He went on a low-fat diet and started walking every day. His wife, Mary, went along to keep him company. After they had worked up from a few blocks to more than five miles a day, they decided to join a local race-walking group. At first they were happy just to complete their events. Then they began to set higher goals, and soon they were winning medals for their age group. They discovered that the other race-walkers were interesting, congenial people who were not content just to sit in front of their television sets. With their newfound friends they started going to races in other cities, and then to international events. Each year they arrange their travel plans around the race schedule. When I last saw Bob and Mary, they were heading off to Japan for a major race. He said, "If you told me fifteen years ago that exercise would become a central passion in my life, I never would have believed you." Bob celebrated his eightieth birthday this year.

The previous chapters have focused on how your diet affects your health and appearance, and how to improve your life with low-fat eating. Adding exercise to your dietary program can make you *look* better by giving you strong muscles and a trim body, and make you *feel* better by increasing brain levels of neurotransmitters that raise your mood.

When you exercise regularly, your heart becomes stronger, so you have greater endurance. Your skeletal muscles become stronger, so you have more strength. Your blood level of the heart-attack-preventing HDL cholesterol rises. If you have high blood pressure, exercise can help to lower it. If you are overweight, exercise will help you burn calories and convert fat to muscle.

This chapter will teach you how to apply the training principles used by world-class athletes to your exercise program. You don't need to exercise as much or as intensely as they do, but you can benefit from the lessons they have learned. Chapter 11 will help you select activities you enjoy and show you how to apply these principles to them.

Exercise Basics

Any kind of exercise is better than no exercise at all. But for cardiovascular fitness and weight loss, your exercise program should be:

- **Aerobic.** Exercise is aerobic if you move continuously for twenty minutes or more.
- **Intense.** You won't get much benefit if you shuffle through your exercise. You need to work hard enough to raise your pulse.
- **Regular.** You should exercise at least three times a week. Five days of alternating sports or activities is even better.

How Exercise Helps You Lose Weight

Most people understand that you burn more calories when you exercise than when you are inactive. You may not realize that exercise also causes you to burn more calories for the rest of the day. Every time you exercise vigorously, your body temperature rises and stays elevated for up to eighteen hours. Swimming is the only exercise that does not give you this benefit, because water conducts heat away from your body. All exercise on land will increase your metabolism because air is a good insulator and your temperature will rise with any vigorous activity.

Exercise also helps you lose weight and keep it off because muscles burn more energy than fat. Muscles are heavier than fat, so if you exercise a lot, don't be surprised if your scales don't show as much of a loss as you expect. Use your tape measure and your eyes to measure your success.

How Exercise Makes You Feel Good

It's called runner's high, but you can get it from any exercise. Vigorous activity makes you feel good, and nobody knows exactly why. One theory is that exercise raises blood levels of endorphins, morphine-like chemicals in your brain; or serotonin or norepinephrine, neurotransmitters that send messages from one nerve to another. Whatever the cause, the good feeling lasts less than a day, so you need to exercise regularly to enjoy the benefits. Vigorous activity also helps you sleep better, so you awaken feeling refreshed.

Starting a New Exercise Program

More than 65 percent of people who start an exercise program drop out within six weeks, usually because of injuries. It took years for your body to get out of shape, and you won't become fit overnight. Be patient. Go slowly and cautiously. You're trying to develop an exercise plan that you can live with for the rest of your life.

The key to exercising safely is to stop exercising when you feel pain in one part of your body. Many people feel pain in their muscles after exercising for just a few minutes. With aging, muscles lose their elasticity and can start to tear very quickly. If you stop exercising as soon as you start to feel discomfort, you are not likely to injure yourself.

Unfortunately, if you stop exercising when you feel local discomfort, you may not be able to exercise long enough to become fit. However, if you exercise for thirty seconds, then rest for thirty seconds, and alternate exercising and resting, you should be able to exercise far longer without injuring yourself. Build up gradually and you can avoid injury.

Stress and Recover

You improve in sports by stressing your muscles and then waiting for them to recover before you stress them again. When you exercise, your muscle fibers are injured — there is bleeding into the fibers and disruption of the Z bands that hold muscle filaments together. If you stress your muscles again while they are still recovering from a previous hard workout, you can tear them, and then you won't be able to exercise at all. On the other hand, if you rest by taking the day off or exercising other muscle groups, the stressed muscles heal and are stronger than they were before you took your hard workout. Most athletes wait at least forty-eight hours to recover before they exercise intensely again. You should wait at least that long also.

Stress refers to how *hard* you exercise, not how *much*. For example, competitive runners run very fast one to three times a week. They can run twenty miles on an easy day, as long as they do it at a much slower pace. Weight lifters lift very heavy weights only once a week. They lift lighter weights with fewer repetitions in the rest of their workouts.

How Much Is Too Much?

Exercise is supposed to make you feel good. If you don't feel good *after* you finish exercising, you're probably exercising *too much*. There's a proper dose for everything. If you don't get enough sleep, you feel tired all the time. If you get too much sleep, you can develop a headache and feel awful. This also applies to eating. If you don't get enough food, you feel hungry. If you eat too much food, you feel sick.

It's the same with exercise. If you get the right amount of exercise, your muscles will feel wonderfully tired, your mood will be good and you will want to pursue other interests. When you exercise too much, you often feel irritated. Your joints, muscles, tendons and bones ache. You don't look forward to exercising again. Your lymph nodes may swell and you may develop frequent infections and injuries.

If you want to enjoy exercising, fit a reasonable program into your schedule and don't do much more. Thirty minutes three times a week is plenty. Remember, thirty minutes of intense exercise is much more worthwhile than hours of just lollygagging along. Many people feel best when they exercise every other day. That allows enough time for their muscles to recover. If you want to exercise *more* often than every other day, alternate sports that use different muscles and listen to your body. If you don't feel like exercising on a particular day, take the day off. Your body is telling you something.

Alternating Sports

Stephanie K. tried to start a running program but couldn't last for more than a mile. She was basically healthy and couldn't understand her lack of progress. She was running five days a week until her legs felt tired, usually after about fifteen minutes. I told her to try running three days a week and cycling on two. I instructed her to run slowly on Monday and Wednesday until her legs felt heavy or sore, and to pedal a bicycle slowly on Tuesday and Thursday. On Fridays she was to run a half mile very slowly to warm up and then do a series of very fast runs for fifteen seconds each followed by slow jogging until she recovered. She was to alternate these fast and slow runs until her legs felt tired. Stephanie followed the program faithfully, and three months later she ran a 10-kilometer race (6.1 miles) in 63 minutes.

When you alternate sports that stress different parts of your body on consecutive days, you make better progress than when you try to do the same activity every day. For example, you can walk (lower leg) on Monday, Wednesday and Friday and row (upper body) on Tuesday and Thursday. You might alternate jogging (lower leg) and swimming (upper body) or aerobic dancing (lower leg) and cycling (upper leg) or cross-country ski machine (upper leg) and pretending to conduct an orchestra (upper body).

Table 9 (page 94) lists sports by the primary parts of your body that each one stresses. From the table, you will see that running, walking and dancing stress primarily the lower leg muscles. Your foot strikes the ground with great force, which is transmitted primarily to your foot and lower leg. Cycling, skating and skiing stress primarily the upper leg mus-

Table 9. Stressing Different Parts of Your Body

Sports That Stress Primarily the Lower Leg	Sports That Stress Primarily the Upper Leg	Sports That Stress Primarily the Upper Body
Running	Cycling	Rowing
Walking	Skiing	Swimming
Dancing	Skating	Hitting a punching bag
		Conducting an orchestra

A Sample Schedule for Alternating Sports

	Program 1	Program 2	Program 3
Mon (easy)	Walk	Jog	Dance
Tue (hard)	Row	Swim	Cycle
Wed (easy)	Walk	Jog	Dance
Thu (easy)	Row	Swim	Cycle
Fri (hard)	Walk	Jog	Dance
Saturday	Off	Off	Off
Sunday	Off	Off	Off

cles because you pedal with your knees and hips and skate and ski by pushing from your hips. Rowing and swimming stress primarily your upper body and back because you pull on the oars with your arms and back, and you drive yourself forward in swimming with your arms, not your legs. Table 9 gives three possible programs and shows how you can schedule one hard day in each activity, with plenty of time for recovery.

Intensity

Competitive athletes train at almost their maximum heart rate, the fastest their heart can beat and still pump blood through their body. They become so short of breath that they can't even talk while they're working out. You don't need to train that hard. First, it hurts and second, training that intensely increases markedly your chances of injuring yourself. To achieve a high level of fitness, all you have to do is exercise intensely enough to increase your need for oxygen to the point where you start to raise your shoulders and start to breathe more frequently, but you still should be able to talk. This will usually raise your pulse to more than 100 beats a minute.

The more *intensely* you exercise, the less time you need to exercise to be fit. For example, you can become more fit by running a couple of miles very fast than by running ten miles very slowly. However, since intense exercise increases your chances of injury, don't pick up the pace more often than *once or twice a week*.

Why Exercise Intensely?

When you run, you burn 100 calories a mile, regardless of whether you run fast or slowly. You keep the same form running fast or slowly, so you use the same motions and you burn the same number of calories a mile. In one study, a group of men ran two miles slowly in twenty-five minutes and burned 200 calories during exercise, while another group ran two miles fast in seventeen minutes and burned the same 200 calories during exercise. The faster group lost far more fat because they increased their metabolism.

Exercising at a very low intensity does not increase your metabolism significantly. To use exercise for weight reduction, you should exercise more intensely. The *harder* you exercise, the greater the increase in your metabolism. You need to exercise to at least 40 percent of your capacity for an exercise session to increase your metabolism significantly. If you exercise at 70 percent of your capacity, you will increase your metabolism seven times more than when you work at 40 percent. That's a tremendous difference in calories burnt and fat lost.

Pulse Rate Measures Intensity

You can use your pulse rate to measure how intensely you exercise. To become more fit, you need to increase your heart rate by more than twenty beats a minute above your resting heart rate.

Most exercise books and instructors tell you to exercise hard enough to raise your pulse rate to 60 percent of your maximum heart rate. This formula is of little practical value and is based on faulty science. Your maximum heart rate is the fastest your heart can beat and still pump blood through your body. It usually comes close to the formula 220 minus your age. As you age, your skeletal muscles weaken, and you can't exercise as intensely as you could when you were younger. Your maximum heart rate is determined by *how hard you can exercise your skeletal muscles*. Your skeletal muscles drive your heart, rather than the other way around. So the maximum-heart-rate concept is really a measure of how strong your muscles are. It is not a measure of heart strength.

You don't need to take your pulse. You can tell when you are exercising intensely because you breathe harder and perspire. You reach your *training heart rate* at the point where you just start to require more oxygen.

Start off slowly, and gradually increase the pace until you start to raise your shoulders and breathe faster to take in more air. You should still be able to talk.

Muscle Burn and Intensity

You can gauge the severity of stress by the amount of burning in your muscles you feel during exercise. If you slow down or stop when you feel burning and heaviness, you will probably be able to exercise on the next day. However, you will not increase your level of fitness very much.

On the other hand, if you keep on pushing through the burning and heaviness, you will probably feel dead-legged for the next one to three days. You should then take the next day or two off or work out at a slow pace until the heaviness goes away. You will be far more fit than the person who does the same low-intensity workout every day.

Muscle Soreness the Day After You Exercise

If you're exercising properly, you can expect your muscles to feel sore on the day after you exercise intensely. The soreness is caused by damage to the muscle fibers. If you don't feel sore the next day, you won't become stronger and faster, and you won't increase your endurance.

If you are satisfied with your level of fitness and feel no need to improve, you can prevent muscle soreness just by stopping exercise when you feel the burning. However, if you're exercising to increase your endurance, you should continue exercising during a workout when your muscles start to burn. Then allow at least forty-eight hours for your muscles to recover before you exercise them again.

Good Muscle Burn or Injury?

How can you tell the difference between the "good" burn of hard exercise and the "bad" pain of an impending injury?

The helpful burning of intense exercise usually occurs in the same muscles on both sides of your body, and the amount of discomfort remains the same as you continue to exercise. When a muscle, ligament or tendon starts to tear, the pain usually occurs on one side only and becomes progressively more severe if you continue the same movement. If you feel that type of pain, stop immediately and try again in a day or two.

How Long Should You Exercise?

You should start out by exercising only until your muscles feel heavy or hurt, and then you should quit for the day. Eventually, try to work up to being able to exercise for thirty minutes. However, *stopping* exercise as soon as you start to feel local discomfort can prevent you from becoming fit. If you can't exercise for thirty minutes continuously in one sport, try to get at least thirty minutes *total* exercise or vigorous activity during the day. Competitive athletes use interval training and so can you. You can apply the concept of interval training:

◆ In one sport
◆ In two or more sports that use different muscle groups

Intervals

Almost 80 percent of American adults can't exercise vigorously or long enough to achieve moderate fitness, so many feel that they will waste their time exercising. According to the American College of Sports Medicine, you don't have to engage in vigorous exercise *for sustained periods* to gain substantial health benefits.[40] If you exercise for thirty seconds, stop for thirty seconds and alternate exercising and resting, you should be able to increase your exercise time without much discomfort and without injuring yourself. An example of a typical workout is to start off by pulling on a rowing machine for thirty seconds, resting for thirty seconds and then alternating rowing and resting for several minutes. Stop when your muscles hurt or feel heavy.

That's the concept of *interval training*, and top athletes in all sports use it. More than thirty-five years ago, the Swedish physiologist Per Olof Astrand showed that you can increase your exercise load markedly by alternating exercise with rest periods.[41] He showed that you could exercise for thirty seconds intensely and continuously without accumulating much lactic acid in your bloodstream. Lactic acid makes muscles hurt and tired. However, the amount that accumulates in thirty seconds of hard work is quickly cleared from your bloodstream. Then you can exercise for another short burst. Your muscles get stronger as you build up the number of intervals you can complete.

You Recover Faster by Resting

Sore muscles recover faster when you take the day off than when you exercise at a leisurely pace. A major source of energy for your muscles is the sugar, called glycogen, that is stored in them. When you exercise vigorously, your muscles use up most of their stored sugar. A low level of stored muscle sugar causes heaviness, weakness and tiredness. Your muscles fill up with stored sugar *faster* while you rest than while you exercise. You would expect this to happen because additional exercise uses up more stored sugar. When you wake up with sore and tired muscles on the day after you have exercised vigorously, take the day off. You deserve it.

Getting Started

It's always a good idea to get your doctor's OK before you start a major new exercise program, particularly if you are overweight or haven't exercised in years. You need to be especially cautious if you are over 40. Once your doctor gives the OK, the next step is to pick an activity you will enjoy, or at least not find too distasteful. You have lots of choices. You can walk, run or ride a bicycle outdoors. You can jog in place or dance to an aerobic videotape in your living room. Investing in a piece of exercise equipment such as a stationary bicycle, treadmill, mini-trampoline or rowing machine may provide the motivation you need. Or you can join an aerobic exercise class. Sports that involve continuous motion — racquetball, handball, rowing, swimming, ice skating, roller-blading — are excellent choices if you have (or can develop) enough skill to get a good aerobic workout. My recommendations for specific sports and exercise equipment are listed in the next chapter.

Select two activities or sports that stress different parts of your body. Start out the first day of your program by exercising at a relaxed pace until your muscles feel heavy or begin to hurt, or until you feel tired. Then stop immediately. If you're over 40 and haven't exercised in more than a year, it may be several weeks before you can exercise for just ten minutes. Gradually, your muscles will get stronger and you will be able to work up to a full thirty minutes.

You may hate every minute of every exercise session at first. But I predict that you'll be gratified by your progress. If you can stick to your program through the first six weeks, you'll find that the rewards are worth it. When you make exercise a part of your life, you'll wonder how you ever got along without it.

Warming Up

Always start each workout at a very low intensity. Putting great force on a cold, resting muscle increases your chances of tearing it. When you exercise, your muscles use chemical reactions to convert foodstuffs to energy. Less than 30 percent of the energy is used to power your muscles. More than 70 percent of the energy is lost as heat. So muscle temperature rises whenever you exercise. Resting muscle temperature is around 98 degrees. After you jog slowly for just a few minutes, your muscle temperature can be as high as 101 degrees, which makes the muscles more pliable and resistant to injury. Warming up also increases the force that your muscles can exert, so you can jump higher, run faster, lift heavier and throw farther.

You could warm up your muscles by taking a warm bath. However, exercising is better because it also increases the blood flow to the muscles you use. Warming up is specific. The best way to warm up for running is to run slowly, and the best way to warm up for swimming is to swim slowly. To prevent injury, you need to warm up for only one to three minutes. To develop maximum power, you need to warm up until you start to sweat and your body temperature rises 1 to 2 degrees.

What's the Best Time to Exercise?

It doesn't really matter when you exercise. You can exercise at any time that suits your schedule, but the best time for many people is before they need to concentrate and think clearly. For four to six hours after you finish exercising, your body temperature remains elevated, your heart pumps more blood and you are more alert.

In one study, schoolchildren were divided into two groups. One group exercised during the lunch break, and the other group just ate lunch. When the children went back to class in the afternoon, those who exercised were able to concentrate and learn more efficiently than those who didn't exercise. Studies on office workers have come up with similar results.

Your mother probably told you not to exercise right after a meal, but most people can exercise after eating without suffering from stomach cramps. Exercising with food in your stomach causes your stomach and skeletal muscles to work hard simultaneously, so they both need large amounts of oxygen. Blood can be shunted to your skeletal muscles and away from your stomach muscles, causing stomach muscles to go into spasm and hurt. If you exercise at a slow pace, your heart should be strong enough to pump blood to both your stomach and your skeletal muscles. If you do get a cramp, just stop and rest.

Treating an Injury

Muscle pulls are a hazard of exercising. The immediate treatment is **RICE: R**est, **I**ce, **C**ompression and **E**levation. Stop exercising immediately, apply an ice bag wrapped in a towel to the injured part, wrap a bandage loosely over the ice bag, and raise the injured part above the heart. Remove the ice after fifteen minutes and reapply it once an hour for the first few hours.

The only drugs that have been shown to help heal muscles are anabolic steroids and beta agonist asthma medications such as clenbutarol or albuterol. Anabolic steroids are illegal and have dangerous side effects. Clenbutarol and albuterol appear to be safe in the low doses that are required to hasten muscle healing, but they have not been approved for use in the United States. It's all right to take pain medicines such as ibuprofen, but they do not speed healing. You may make matters worse if you mask the pain that warns you not to use the injured muscle. Cortisone-type injections block pain and reduce swelling, but they may actually delay healing.

In the long term, the only effective treatment is rest. You should not exercise that part of your body until you can do so without feeling pain. When you return to exercising, start out at reduced intensity and duration, working back up gradually to your normal load. Stop immediately if you feel pain.

> **Patty L.** wanted help with a foot injury so she could get back to the running she loved. She was tall, muscular and weighed 142 pounds. It was hard to believe that she was the same person as the one in a photograph she showed me. Five years before, she had weighed 240 pounds. She told me she had started counting fat grams and exercising after hearing my radio program, lost 90 pounds in eighteen months, and kept the weight off even after having a child. Now she runs races regularly and was terribly frustrated by her injury. I told her to listen to her body and not run again until the pain was completely gone, but she could ride a bicycle in the meantime. Two sports are always better than one.

Extra Precautions if You're Over 50

When older people damage their muscles during exercise, they heal just as quickly as younger people do. Most older people will find this hard to believe. In one study, older people recovered from vigorous exercise just as rapidly as college students. However, they have to exercise less frequently and with less intensity because:

- ◆ **They have fewer muscle fibers**
- ◆ **The remaining fibers lose some of their elasticity**

Your muscles lose fibers. Muscles are made up of thousands of individual fibers, just as a rope is made up of many smaller threads. Each muscle fiber is innervated by a single nerve. As you age, your nerves start to die and disappear. When you lose nerves, you also lose function in the muscle fiber innervated by that nerve (Figure 8). Thus, older people have fewer fibers in their muscles and are more likely to injure themselves when they try to take the same workout as a younger person.

The good news is that your remaining muscle fibers are just as trainable as when you were younger, so you can become stronger and faster and

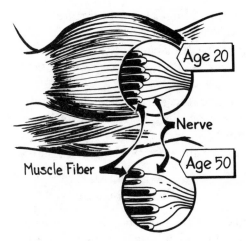

Fig. 8. *A single nerve goes to each muscle fiber.*

With aging, nerves die. When a nerve dies, the muscle fiber stops functioning. Older people have fewer working muscle fibers, so they injure more easily.

increase your endurance as long as you stop exercising when you feel pain.

Your muscles lose elasticity. When you are young, your muscles and tendons stretch and contract like rubber bands. As you age, your tendons and muscles lose their springiness and become more brittle and likely to tear. This can affect the way you exercise and even the way that you walk. When you walk, your heel strikes the ground with a force equal to most of your own weight, causing your muscles to contract and stretch their tendons. More than two-thirds of the force of your footstrike is stored in the tendons as they are stretched. Then when you move forward onto your toes, the tendons snap back and release the stored energy to drive you forward (Figure 9). With aging, your tendons can't store as much energy without tearing, so you take shorter steps when you walk and run. This slows you down and can make you look awkward.

Taking such small strides does not require much use of your upper leg muscles, which causes them to weaken. More than 80 percent of people over 70 can't get out of a chair without using their hands, and they can't

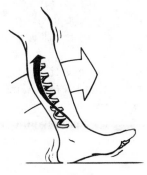

Fig. 9. *Tendons lose their springiness with age. You take shorter steps and your leg muscles get weaker.*

walk up stairs without holding on to the railing. They can strengthen the upper leg muscles by pedaling a bicycle, skiing, skating or walking uphill.

Eighty-five percent of older people have back pain mostly because they have osteoporosis and weak back muscles. Both can be prevented and treated with back-strengthening exercises.

The best exercise program to retard the effects of aging includes strengthening your upper leg muscles by pedaling a recumbent stationary bicycle on one day and strengthening your back muscles by pulling on a rowing machine on the next. If you feel pain or fatigue, stop immediately and try again the next day.

Many Markers of Aging Are Really Markers of Fitness

Many older people won't exercise because they feel that they are too old to become stronger, and they are afraid of injuring themselves. Most healthy older people can triple their strength in a few months just by lifting weights. You need to exercise when you are older even more than you did when you were young.

Doctors often determine how our bodies age by measuring our VO_2max, the maximal amount of oxygen that a person can take in and use. Studies show that older men who continue to train and compete in long-distance running races are able to maintain their VO_2max. This is astounding. It means that a test that doctors use to measure aging may actually be measuring fitness, and that much of the aging and decline in quality of life that accompanies aging may be caused more by inactivity than by aging itself.

Any Exercise Is Better Than No Exercise

To reach your thirty-minute total of exercise or vigorous activity during the day, you can use several different sports or activities and stop exercising when you feel the least discomfort. Resume exercise in another activity when you have recovered. For example, go to an aerobic dance class and stop when you feel the least bit tired, even if you have to quit after two minutes. Rest, and then ride a stationary bike until your legs start to feel heavy, perhaps for three minutes. Later in the day, walk for a short distance until you feel tired.

Try for a combined total time of thirty minutes of exercise a day, five days a week. You can count any physical activity that keeps you moving constantly, such as walking, climbing stairs, mopping floors or gardening. The next chapter is full of suggestions for exercises you may enjoy.

CHAPTER 11

Choose Your Sports!

People often ask me what is the best exercise. The answer is, any activity that can raise your pulse above 90 beats a minute and keep it there for ten to thirty minutes. Tennis and golf may be a lot of fun, but they don't meet my definition of exercise. Unless you are up with the pros, you spend more time on the tennis court waiting for the ball than you do moving. And no matter how good a golfer you are, the leisurely pace of the game makes it ineffective as exercise.

Choose one or two activities from Table 10. If you've been inactive for a long time or have health problems, fast walking and riding a recumbent stationary bicycle are probably your best choices. When you take up a

Table 10. Good Exercises for Fitness

Aerobic dancing	*Vigorous Use of Exercise Equipment*
Cross-country skiing	Cross-country ski machine
Cycling	Mini-trampoline
Dancing (continuous)	Recumbent stationary bicycle
Fast walking	Rowing machine
Handball	Stair-stepper
Ice-skating	Stationary bicycle
Jogging	Treadmill
Racquetball	
Rollerblading	
Rowing	
Running	
Squash	
Step aerobics	
Swimming	

new sport, remember that it will take time to develop enough skill so you can sustain your training pulse and exercise safely.

Don't scrimp on proper equipment for the activity you select. Good shoes are essential for walking, jogging, running and aerobics. Bicycling requires a helmet, and rollerbladers need knee and elbow pads. If you invest in an exercise machine to use in your home, make sure it is sturdy and smooth-running.

Easy Exercises

If you are starting your first exercise program or if you haven't exercised in a long time, pick an activity that's easy to do. You can build up your level of fitness without having to learn any new skills, and you will be much less likely to injure yourself in the first few weeks. Here are the exercises that I recommend.

Fast Walking

Walking is a safe sport because it rarely causes injuries. Running causes injuries frequently because you take both feet off the ground at the same time and land with a tremendous force that can tear muscles and shatter bones. On the other hand, when you walk, you always keep at least one foot on the ground and land with minimal footstrike force. However, if you want to walk to become fit, you have to move fast. You should exercise vigorously enough to increase your heart rate at least 20 beats a minute higher than when you rest. That means you will be breathing harder and perspiring.

There are two ways to increase your walking speed. You can take longer steps or you can move your feet at a faster rate. To lengthen your stride, swivel your hips so you reach farther forward with your feet. This will cause you to twist your body from side to side, which will tend to make you point your toes inward when your feet touch the ground. When you point in, you lose distance. Try to point your toes forward with each step.

To move your feet at a faster rate, you have to move your arms faster. Every time you move one leg forward, you pull the arm on the same side back and the arm on the other side moves forward. Your legs will only move as fast as you can move your arms.

Bend your elbows so you can move your arms faster. The fulcrum of your arm-swing is at your shoulder. The straighter you keep your elbows, the longer it takes your arms to swing forward and back. Bending your elbows shortens the swing and helps you move faster.

Stationary Bicycle

Riding a stationary bicycle is an excellent low-risk exercise. The large muscles of your legs get a vigorous workout, and the smooth rotary motion of pedaling is easy on your joints.

Start out by pedaling at the lowest resistance until your legs feel tired or start to hurt. Gradually work up to thirty minutes of continuous cycling every other day. When you can do this, start working on intensity.

Warm up for a few minutes, then set the pedal tension slightly higher. Pedal until you feel tired, then lower the resistance again. When you can get through your entire thirty minutes with the tension raised, set it a little higher. At the same time, spend part of your workout pedaling a little faster. As your fitness improves, keep increasing your speed and resistance in increments. Before long, you will be getting a very intense workout.

If you decide to buy a stationary bike, find one that pedals smoothly as you increase the tension. Get one with straps on the pedals to help you keep your feet in place. While you're shopping, be sure to try a recumbent bicycle that has pedals at the same height as your hips. That's what I use.

Recumbent Stationary Bicycle

People who find a regular stationary bicycle uncomfortable may prefer a recumbent bicycle. With a regular stationary bicycle, you sit on a narrow seat to allow your legs to reach down to the pedals. The seat can press your pudendal nerve against your pelvic bones and cause numbness and pain. On the other hand, on a recumbent bicycle, your legs are at the same level as your hips, so you don't need a narrow seat. You sit in a contoured chair that does not exert any pressure against your pelvis. It also supports your back.

As with a regular stationary bicycle, you pedal against slight resistance at a comfortable speed until your legs feel heavy or until they hurt. Do this every other day until you can pedal for ten to twenty minutes. Then gradually increase your speed and resistance.

A recumbent bicycle is ideal for older people. Most people over 60 have extraordinarily weak upper leg muscles. If you can't walk up stairs without holding on and can't raise yourself from a chair without using your hands, you can increase your upper leg strength by pedaling a bicycle. Older people who would have difficulty balancing on a regular stationary bicycle will have no problem using a recumbent model. Recumbent bicycles also make exercise possible for many people with special health problems. Virtually anyone who can sit in a chair can use one.

Aerobic Dancing

Aerobic dance classes are offered in most communities and are deservedly popular. Aerobics use your whole body. You can work at your own level with guidance from an experienced instructor. Lively music and familiar routines make your workout fun. Committing yourself to a class schedule and getting together with friends can help to keep you motivated.

You will need shoes that give you good support around the heel and absorb the shock of your foot striking the floor. Shoes designed for aerobic dancing allow you to move from side to side as well as forward.

Low-impact aerobics eliminate the jumping and pounding of regular aerobic dancing. You keep one foot on the floor at all times and move up and down by bending and straightening your knees, so there is less stress on your joints.

Whether you do high- or low-impact aerobics, your goal will be thirty minutes of sustained dancing at your training pulse rate, plus warm-up and cool-down periods. Most instructors do periodic pulse checks to help you monitor your progress. You can also do aerobic dancing at home using one of the many videotapes on the market.

Step Aerobics

In this variation on aerobic dancing, participants use a low platform and add up-and-down stepping motions to their routines. You can use the same principle at home. Step aerobics are good exercise, and you don't need expensive equipment.

A 6- to 10-inch step is ideal. Step up with one foot, then the other, then down with your first foot and down with the second. Do this every other day until your legs feel heavy or until they hurt. You use the muscles in your upper legs to raise yourself up on a step, and these muscles tire very easily. In the beginning, you probably won't be able to go up and down for more than a few minutes at a time. Gradually, your "quad" and hamstring muscles will become stronger, and you will be able to work up to twenty or thirty minutes. Then try to go faster. You don't have to spend more time.

Jogging on a Mini-trampoline

A mini-trampoline gives you the aerobic benefits of jogging with much less stress on your joints. The trampoline mat gives with each step you take, so the force of your footstrike is about one-sixth of what it would be on hard pavement. Since you use the trampoline at home, you can always stop when you get tired or sore.

Start out slowly until you are sure of your balance. You can simulate walking at a brisk pace, then gradually increase your speed.

Rowing Machines

Rowing is excellent exercise because it uses the large muscles of your legs and back as well as your arms. All good rowing machines have moving seats. When you row, bring your seat forward as far as possible. Start rowing by pushing your feet against the stirrups so the seat starts to move backward. When the seat starts to move, lean back. Then finish up by pulling the oars close to your body.

The best type of rowing machine on the market has a spinning wheel. You pull on oars that are attached to a rope that causes the wheel to spin. Since the rate at which the wheel spins is a function of how hard you pull on the handles, you can accelerate and decelerate as you pull. Tension on the wheel can be increased gradually as you get stronger.

Stair-Steppers

A stair-stepper machine can give you the same workout you'd get running up the steps of the Washington Monument. And since your feet stay in one place, you don't pound and cause a lot of stress on your joints. However, you do need to be careful when you use a stair-climber. If you step too deeply, you can hurt your knees. Take only small steps of 4 to 6 inches; keep your entire foot on the pedal and don't try to rise up on your toes. When you step on the pedals, keep your back straight and use the handles to balance yourself. Don't lean forward or put your weight on your hands. You want to keep your center of gravity over the pedals to prevent back pain.

You work against gravity on a stair-stepper, so the weight of your own body provides some resistance, just as it does when you climb uphill. As you get stronger, you can adjust the machine to add more resistance or accelerate your pace.

Cross-Country Ski Machines

Moving like a cross-country skier exercises both your legs and your upper body. You may enjoy using a ski machine such as NordicTrack, or you may find the motions difficult to master. Cross-country ski machines require more coordination than the other types of exercise equipment I've described. Be sure to try one out before you buy.

Swimming

Swimming works your whole body — legs, arms and back. Swimming is easy on the joints and is often recommended as an exercise for people with health problems. You can swim at your own rate and use any stroke you like. To get aerobic benefit from swimming, you need to do more than paddle around the pool. Work up gradually to thirty minutes of continuous swimming.

If weight loss is your primary goal, swimming is not as effective as exercising on land. Your body temperature rises when you exercise on land because air is a good insulator, so your metabolism stays elevated after you finish. When you swim, water conducts heat away from your body so that your temperature does not rise and you don't get the benefit of increased metabolism.

Skills and Sports

When you can get through a thirty-minute workout at your training pulse rate with no trouble, you may want to add some variety to your exercise program. You can take up an activity you enjoyed when you were younger, or you can learn a new sport. The following sports and exercises need at least a moderate level of fitness and some skill. They also have a higher risk of injury.

Jogging and Running

If you think you would enjoy jogging or running, here's how to get started. First, check with your doctor and get a good pair of running shoes. Start out by jogging slowly until your legs feel heavy or start to hurt or until you feel tired. Then stop for the day, even if you have taken only a few steps. Do this every day or every other day. You should be able to work up to the point where you can jog slowly for at least twenty minutes. If you're happy with this program, you don't have to go any further. However, if you want to improve, follow the training methods that competitive runners use.

On one day, start out slowly and gradually pick up the pace. When you start to feel uncomfortable, slow down. When you recover, pick up the pace again. On the next day, if your legs feel stiff, don't try to run. If you feel all right, run very slowly. Try to do these gradual pickup workouts every other day. Never do them when your legs are stiff or tired.

After a few months of alternating days of pickups and slow runs, you are ready to take the next step: intervals and longer runs. On Tuesdays and Thursdays, run faster. On Tuesday, try to run 220 yards fast (half a track length), jog very slowly for the same distance, and then repeat the 220-yard runs until your legs start to feel stiff. On Thursday, try to run two to five miles fairly fast, and on Sunday, try to increase your distance so you can run for at least an hour. On the other days, either run slowly or, if your legs feel stiff, take the day off.

How to Use a Treadmill

Most people prefer to walk, jog or run outdoors, but what do you do when the weather is cold and wet or it's dark outside? You may want to consider a treadmill.

Don't buy a treadmill unless it has at least a one-horsepower motor and can attain a speed of at least seven miles an hour. If the motor is weaker than that, the force of your footstrike can overcome the speed of the treadmill, and it will turn with a jerky motion. You don't need a lot of gadgets; they won't give you a better workout.

Never get on a treadmill unless you're wearing good running shoes. Your feet strike the belt with great force and then turn inward. Good running shoes prevent injuries by dampening the footstrike force and limiting inward rolling of your feet.

Start out with a speed lower than two miles an hour to allow time for your muscles to warm up. After you start to sweat, you are warmed up and can move faster. Do not increase the speed by more than a half mile an hour each couple of minutes.

To increase your level of fitness, you need to increase the intensity of your runs. With this regimen, you will increase your speed by one mile an hour every four minutes. Slow down when you feel short of breath, and stop if you feel pain or discomfort. Try again two days later with the same regimen. Remember, in the first six weeks of a new exercise, it's better to stop too early than too late.

Bicycling

If you rode a bicycle as a child, you can probably ride one now. You may be a little shaky at first, but the skill will come back with practice. Borrow or rent a bike and try it out. Always wear a helmet. Without one, a minor fall can result in a serious head injury.

Cycling is excellent exercise because it uses the large muscles of your upper legs, and the smooth rotary motion doesn't pound your joints. If you enjoy riding and have access to bike trails or lightly traveled roads, you will soon be shopping for a good bicycle: a racing bike if you're competitive, a mountain bike if you'll be riding mainly on trails or a touring bicycle if you just want to wander around country back roads.

Most communities have cycling clubs that organize rides and social events. Check with a local bicycle shop or write the League of American Bicyclists, P.O. Box 988, Baltimore, MD 21203.

Riding a Tandem Bicycle

If you are in much better shape than your mate, you still can exercise together when you ride a tandem bicycle. A regular bicycle rider in good shape can spin the pedals more than eighty times a minute. A beginner may spin them at half that rate. When you ride a tandem together, both of you will spin at the faster cadence and both will get a good workout. If one person puts twice as much pressure on the pedals, that person gets twice as much exercise.

The more experienced rider sits in the front seat. The person who sits in the back (the stoker) just pedals, while the front rider (the captain) does the steering, shifting and braking. The captain needs to tell the stoker about upcoming bumps, stops or gear changes. You may have to stand up when you go uphill. The stoker stands first while the captain keeps the bike stable; then a few seconds later, the captain can stand up, too.

Many bicycle shops will give you instructions and let you take a trial ride on a tandem. If you try it, I bet you'll love it.

> **Hal C.** won the gold medal for the hammer throw in the 1956 Olympics. When he came to my office in 1993, I couldn't believe it was the same person. I had seen him in Boston when I was in college, and he was huge. Since then, he'd had so many injuries and problems with arthritis in his arms, hips and legs that now he couldn't participate in any sports at all. He was very frustrated because he missed the wonderful feeling he always got from working out. I invited him to try riding a tandem bicycle with us. The rotary motion of pedaling doesn't put much stress on hips, knees and other joints the way lots of other sports do, and he wouldn't have to worry about coordination if someone else rode in the front. His wife is also very athletic and was able to control the steering, shifting and braking, so all Hal had to do was pedal. They enjoyed it but weren't very stable on our bike because it didn't fit them. When they bought their own bike, they were able to get special handlebars that let Hal sit comfortably. Now they can ride as hard as they like without aggravating his injuries, and they both get a great workout.

Skating

Rollerblading is great exercise if you are reasonably well coordinated and have access to open roads or trails where you can skate continuously for thirty minutes. If you decide to take up this popular sport, get all the recommended protective padding. Find an experienced skater to show you how to stop and turn. Practice in an open parking lot before you take to the road. It may take a while to develop enough skill to sustain your training pulse rate.

Ice-skating also requires considerable skill to qualify as a fitness exercise. You need to skate continuously around the rink fast enough to raise your pulse. Doing figures in the middle of the rink doesn't count.

Racquetball, Handball and Squash

Racquetball is an intensely competitive game that requires much less skill than tennis. All you have to do is hit the ball off any wall or off the ceiling of the court. With basic instruction and a little practice, you'll probably be able to keep the ball in play enough to maintain your training pulse for thirty minutes. The similar sports of handball and squash are equally good exercise if you play hard.

A Word about Weight Training

So far I've talked about aerobic exercises that improve your fitness. Some of them also strengthen specific muscles because you work against resistance. For example, you strengthen your upper leg muscles when you pedal uphill on a bicycle.

Weight training is not an aerobic exercise, but it does have some important benefits. Muscles are made up of thousands of fibers. Each muscle fiber is activated by a single nerve that gets its messages from the brain. As you age, nerve cells wither and die. When a nerve dies, the muscle that is attached to it also dies. With aging, each muscle has fewer fibers to do the same job, so it becomes weaker. To retain strength as you age, you have to enlarge and strengthen the remaining muscle fibers. The only way to do this is to exercise against resistance.

Weight training also strengthens bones. If they live long enough, all women and most men will develop osteoporosis, a condition that weakens bones so they break with even the slightest trauma. Talk to your doctor about your risk for osteoporosis, and include weight training in your program of prevention or treatment.

Lifting a heavy weight causes blood pressure to rise considerably. This can break blood vessels that are already weakened by aging and cause irregular beats in weak hearts. People with normal hearts and blood vessels should not have any problem.

If you want to become stronger, check with your doctor to see if you have any medical problems that will be aggravated by strength training. If you don't, you can join an exercise club and learn how to use weights or special strength-training machines. Or you can purchase a set of weights to use at home. Either way, it's very important to have an experienced instructor show you how to use the equipment. Pick ten to twenty exercises and do them two or three times a week, never on consecutive days. Lift the heaviest weight that you can move comfortably ten times in a row, without straining and without losing form.

I don't recommend the small weights you carry or wear on your wrists or ankles for jogging or aerobic dancing. They interfere with your natural movements, slow you down and don't provide enough resistance to have any real strengthening benefit.

Buying Exercise Equipment

I've talked about what to look for in some of the specific exercise machines you may wish to buy. Here are some general guidelines.

There are lots of advantages to having your favorite piece of exercise equipment in your own home. You can exercise whenever it's convenient, in any weather. You never have to wait in line. You have privacy — a real plus if you're embarrassed about your weight or lack of fitness. You can watch television or listen to music while you exercise.

But good exercise equipment can be expensive. Make sure you know just what you want before you buy. If you have access to a health club or gym, try out the pieces that interest you. It's best to work through the first several weeks of a new exercise program on someone else's machine just to make sure you're comfortable, can master the movements and — hopefully — enjoy the activity. That way you're less likely to end up with a costly machine gathering dust in the basement.

Once you've settled on the type of machine you want, find a store that carries several different models and has them on display so you can try them out. Remember that health clubs buy extremely heavy duty equipment; many machines built for home use are lightweight and poorly constructed. If you buy a machine that doesn't move smoothly, rattles and shakes or fails to give you the range of resistance you need, you won't enjoy your workout.

A good salesperson can explain the special features of each machine and give you rudimentary instruction in its use. You don't necessarily need to buy the most expensive machine — you can do without all the electronic gadgetry. Don't get pressured into something you don't need or want. But do buy the sturdiest, smoothest-operating model you can afford.

If you're thinking about giving exercise equipment as a gift, make sure you know just what the recipient wants. This is not the place for surprises. Ideally you should shop together to check fit and to let the person who will be using the equipment decide which features are most important.

CHAPTER 12

The 50 Most Frequently Asked Questions on My Radio Show

Diet Questions

How can I be sure I'm getting enough protein if I eat mostly fruits, grains, vegetables and beans on a low-fat diet?

Americans get most of their protein from high-fat foods, such as meat, chicken and dairy products made from whole milk. When you go on a low-fat diet, you will eat fewer animal products, but you can get all the protein you need from plants. The main source of low-fat plant protein is beans. Unless you are a strict vegetarian, I recommend that you also use skim milk on your cereal every day and eat seafood 3 to 4 times a week.

You don't need much protein. You get plenty when you eat a cup of skim milk, a cup of breakfast cereal, a cup of beans and a cup of corn or whole grains in a day. It isn't hard to tell if you aren't getting enough; an early sign of protein deficiency is hair loss. However, protein deficiency is virtually unheard of in countries where food is plentiful. Too much protein contributes to osteoporosis.[42]

I'm a vegetarian. How can I be sure I get the right combination of essential amino acids at every meal?

Don't worry about it. Your body cannot absorb whole proteins. Protein is made up of building blocks called amino acids. When you eat protein, your body breaks it down into amino acids, either alone or in small chains. Then when your body needs a protein, it makes the protein anew from the amino acids in your blood and tissues.

There are twenty-two amino acids in your body. Your body requires only nine essential amino acids since it can make the other thirteen from the essential nine. All animal proteins, such as meat, fish, chicken, milk and eggs, contain all nine essential amino acids. However, all plant foods are low in at least one. Vegetarians get all of the amino acids they need by eating a *variety* of foods. If you eat rice, which is low in lysine, and beans, which are low in methionine, you get all nine essential amino acids. But you do not have to eat them together at the same meal or even in the same day.

If any of the nine essential amino acids were missing in your *body*, the entire manufacture of protein in your body would stop. However, every tissue in your body constantly releases amino acids into your bloodstream, and amino acids constantly go back into all tissues. So your blood is loaded with all of the essential amino acids all the time. As long as you eat a variety of beans, vegetables and grains, you don't need to be concerned with specific combinations at each meal.

Does it matter if I eat several small meals rather than three large ones?

The average American eats one-fourth of his of her calories at breakfast, one-fourth at lunch and the remaining half for supper. One study showed that eating the same number of calories in nine meals, rather than three, lowers cholesterol.[43] When the subjects ate every one or two hours, their cholesterol dropped about 6 percent. Since a 1 percent drop in cholesterol equals a 2 percent drop in heart attack risk, nibbling may indeed be more healthful than gorging.

You can lower your cholesterol and lose weight by eating small amounts of food frequently, rather than large amounts a few times a day. Eating raises your temperature for up to four hours. This increases your metabolism so that you burn more calories. If you nibble all day long, you increase your metabolism all day long, so more calories are converted to energy and fewer to fat. Nibbling lowers cholesterol *only* if you don't increase your total intake of food.

Will dieting slow my metabolism?

The most common cause of obesity is a slow metabolic rate that is inherited from your parents. That's why some people are thin even though they eat all day long, while others are fat even though they don't eat a lot.

Dieting slows your metabolism even more. If you eat tiny portions of food and feel hungry all the time, your brain will think you are starving and conserve energy by slowing your metabolism. Calorie-restriction diets don't work. You may lose weight, but you have less than one chance in ten of keeping that weight off one year later. You won't spend the rest of your life feeling hungry when you finish each meal and when you go to bed each night. You will return to your old eating habits, and soon the pounds will creep back on.

My low-fat diet doesn't slow your metabolism because you don't ever feel hungry. The food you eat is full of fiber, and fiber is the only substance that tricks your brain into thinking you are full without contributing any calories.

If you add exercise to your low-fat eating program, you can even speed up your metabolism. Intense exercise increases your body temperature for as much as eighteen hours, so you keep on burning extra calories long after your exercise session is over. Furthermore, muscle burns more calories than fat. As your body changes to more muscle and less fat, you will burn more calories pound for pound.

What about diet pills?

Many entrepreneurs advertise foods, diets, gimmicks, pills and other merchandise they claim will help you lose weight painlessly. The majority are frauds. Various stimulants may suppress your appetite and increase your metabolism slightly, but they may also make you irritable and shaky, interfere with your sleep and raise your blood pressure. You can buy stimulants such as phenylpropanolamine without a prescription; however, you would need to keep increasing the dose, as they lose their effectiveness over time.

Prescription drugs for weight loss affect neurotransmitters, chemicals that carry messages from one nerve to another and control how you think, feel, move your muscles and just about everything else you do. One neurotransmitter, serotonin, helps make you feel full. Another, dopamine, helps to suppress appetite. Some researchers believe that raising the brain levels of these neurotransmitters with a combination of two drugs, fenfluramine and phentermine, can help people lose weight and keep it off. Other researchers cite studies of brain damage in animals from these drugs. You may want to talk with your doctor about the latest findings, but until all the questions about side effects have been answered, I wouldn't recommend them. A permanent change of eating habits combined with exercise is the safest, most effective way to lose weight.

I'm overweight and a friend told me I should take thyroid pills. Will they help me lose weight?

Your thyroid gland secretes a hormone that increases your metabolism, and if it's not doing its job, thyroid pills can help you lose weight. However, taking extra thyroid when your own thyroid gland is giving you the right amount won't cause you to lose weight and can harm you.

All people who are overweight should get a blood test for thyroid function. Until a few years ago, doctors measured just the hormones produced by the thyroid gland. They failed to diagnose many people who had low thyroid function and could have benefited from taking thyroid pills.

Doctors now know that a person can have low thyroid function and still have normal levels of thyroid hormones, if levels of TSH, the hormone produced by the brain, are high. When blood levels of thyroid hormones drop, your brain releases TSH into the bloodstream, which causes the thyroid gland to produce thyroid hormones. Then when your thyroid gland releases thyroid hormones, it keeps the brain from producing too much TSH. In rare cases, high levels of TSH can be caused by a brain tumor. However, the vast majority of people with high blood levels of TSH need to take thyroid pills, even if their blood levels of the thyroid hormones are normal.

Several recent studies show that taking thyroid pills when you *don't* need them can cause osteoporosis, a weakening of bones that markedly increases their chances of being broken.

Can you develop a fat deficiency on a low-fat diet?

You need fat to help you absorb minerals and fat-soluble vitamins. However, it's virtually impossible to be fat deficient unless you are starving. Even if you remove all obvious sources of fat from your diet, you are still eating fat because *all* foods contain some fat, even an apple or a stalk of celery. When foods are labeled 0 grams of fat, that just means they have *less than 1 gram of fat.* No one knows *exactly* how much fat you need, but if you eat 20 grams per day, you will be perfectly healthy. Americans take in, on the average, more than four times that amount, or 85 grams a day.

Is it true that drinking lots of water when you eat will help you lose weight?

Drinking extra water with meals will not reduce the amount of food that you eat. If you drink several glasses of water with your meals, the extra water will distend your stomach and make you feel full for a minute or two, but the water leaves your stomach almost immediately. The only stimulus to make you stop eating is to take in enough food to make you feel full and satisfied. Water does not satisfy hunger.

Healthy kidneys are so effective in clearing extra fluid from your body that you can take in a lot of extra water safely. Your kidneys can clear 5 gallons of water a day or a half glass of water every fifteen minutes. You can drink all the water you like, but don't expect it to help you lose weight. Foods that are high in fiber *will* help because fiber fills you up without contributing any calories. Forget about extra water; eat lots of fruits, vegetables, whole grains and beans.

Will fasting help me lose weight?

Any weight lost while fasting is quickly regained. For permanent weight loss, you need a permanent change in your eating habits. Skipping a few meals won't hurt you, but there are no known health benefits from fasting, and doing it for more than a short time can be harmful. Claims that fasting gives the intestines a rest and helps to clean toxins from the colon are ridiculous. There is no evidence that your intestines need to rest or that toxins from undigested food accumulate in your intestines.

Carried to extreme, fasting can cause problems. Within hours after you start to fast, your body uses up all of its available sugar stored in muscles and liver. Then you have to break down your own body for energy, just as in the movie *The African Queen* Humphrey Bogart dismantles his ship and uses the wood as fuel for his boiler. First, your body uses up all of its stored fat. Then it starts to use your muscles for energy. Your heart is a muscle, and as it is used up, it gets progressively smaller and weaker. The cause of death in starvation is heart failure because the heart becomes too weak to pump blood through the body. The longest a person has been documented to live without food is sixty-six days.

Why do you say liquid diets don't work?

Just ask Oprah Winfrey. The FTC has ordered manufacturers of liquid diets to trim their claims. Drinking 420 to 800 calories a day does take the weight off, but it does not correct the eating habits that caused the weight problem. As soon as the diet is over, the dieter begins to regain the lost weight. Losing weight rapidly can cause gall stones, and regaining weight causes formation of plaques in the arteries. New York City's consumer affairs commissioner proposed a rule requiring weight loss centers to post warnings about the dangers of rapid weight loss along with their drop-out rates. The only way to lose weight permanently is to change your eating habits permanently and get more exercise.

What's the difference between soluble fiber and insoluble fiber?

Fiber is a type of carbohydrate that your body cannot break down, so you can't absorb it. There are two types: soluble and insoluble. Insoluble fiber adds bulk to your stool and helps to prevent constipation. Soluble fiber binds to fat in the intestines and keeps some fat from being absorbed.

Your body needs both kinds of fiber, and they are both found in fruits, vegetables, whole grains and beans. Insoluble fiber may help prevent colorectal cancer by speeding cancer-causing agents through the digestive system. Soluble fiber helps with weight control because its bulk makes you feel full. It can help control diabetes because it slows the rate at which your body absorbs glucose. Soluble fiber has an added benefit. When you add more soluble fiber to your diet, it lowers blood levels of the plaque-forming LDL cholesterol. Soluble fiber is degraded by bacteria in the colon to form types of fatty acids that are absorbed into the bloodstream and help to block the synthesis of cholesterol by the liver. This is the only food component we know that will lower blood cholesterol when you add more to your diet. However, people who have high blood levels of cholesterol must do a lot more than just add soluble fiber to their diet. They also should not smoke or be overweight and should stay on a low-fat diet and exercise regularly.

Questions about Specific Foods and Supplements

How can I tell if a food is high in fat?

Read the labels. Any food that contains more than 2 grams of fat per serving is high in fat. If fat grams are not listed, avoid a food if fats appear on the list of ingredients.

Produce and meats don't have labels, but my rules for these departments of your supermarket are simple. Stay away from the meat counter. Everything in the produce department is fine except avocados, coconuts, nuts, peanuts and soybeans or soybean products, such as tofu.

There's so much information on food labels now. What's important?

Check the grams of fat. You will also want to look at the portion size to make sure it is reasonable. This is all you need to help you stay under 20 grams per day. Ignore the percentage information; it's based on getting 30 *percent* of your calories from fat, and that's way too much. Don't worry about the rest of the information on the label. Counting calories doesn't work, and you don't need to compute your protein, carbohydrates, sodium or vitamins as long as you eat plenty of fruits, vegetables, whole grains and beans.

Please explain what kinds of oils I should eat and which ones I should avoid.

If you're eating *extra* corn, fish or olive oils because you think that they prevent heart attacks, you're taking in a lot of extra calories for the wrong reason. If you want to lower cholesterol or lose weight, you should restrict fats of all kinds.

No oil contains only one type of fat. Corn oil is known primarily for its unsaturated fat content because it contains 57 percent unsaturated fat, but it also contains 30 percent monounsaturated fat and 11 percent saturated fat. Butter is known as a rich source of saturated fat because it contains 69 percent saturated fat, but it also contains 36 percent monounsaturated fat and 3 percent unsaturated fat. Olive oil is known for its monounsaturated fat because it contains 81 percent monounsaturated fat, but it also contains 12 percent saturated fat and 7 percent unsaturated fat.

You don't *need* to eat any kind of oil. If you don't have a problem with your cholesterol or your weight, I would choose an oil that is high in monounsaturated fat, such as olive oil, over the other types.

I thought I only needed to cut out saturated fat to lower my cholesterol.

Saturated fat raises cholesterol more than any other component of your diet, but whenever you eat any kind of fat, you are getting some saturated fat. All natural sources of fats contain monounsaturated, polyunsaturated and saturated fats in various combinations. Restricting all fats lowers cholesterol more than restricting just foods that are high in saturated fat.

The most effective way to reduce high blood levels of cholesterol is to eat less food. A diet with a lot of saturated fat, but with two-thirds of the calories your body needs each day, would lower your cholesterol. Animals and humans eat the most food when they are placed on a cafeteria diet that contains large amounts of fats and sugars. Fats make foods taste so good that you eat more than your body needs. If you eat low-fat foods with lots of fiber, you can reduce your total calories without feeling hungry. That's the best way to lower your cholesterol.

Can I use spray oils on a low-fat diet?

Oil sprays such as Pam add so little fat that you can use them sparingly without counting any extra grams. Even better, you can get the same effect by using nonstick cookware.

What are monoglycerides and diglycerides and should I avoid them?

Monoglycerides and diglycerides are fats that usually occur in foods in such small amounts that you don't have to be concerned about them. Almost all of the fat that you eat is in the form of triglycerides, or "three fats."

Triglycerides have a chemical structure shaped like an E formed by a straight vertical line and three horizontal lines, each comprising a fatty acid. Monoglycerides have the same single vertical line of the E, but they have only one horizontal fatty acid, and diglycerides have two horizontal fatty acids. All three glycerides affect your body in the same way. They have 9 calories per gram and are broken down in the same way to form the same building blocks that are absorbed from your intestines into your bloodstream.

Monoglycerides and diglycerides are added to bakery products to make them taste smooth and to peanut butter to prevent the oil from separating out. They are added in such small amounts that they are insignificant. However, you should look at the *total grams of fat* on the label. Most of the foods with monoglycerides and diglycerides are high-fat foods that you should avoid on a low-fat diet.

Are foods made with the new fat substitutes OK on a low-fat diet?

Pastries, cookies and ice cream made with fat substitutes are low-fiber foods. Even though they are made without fat, they still have a lot of calories. They taste good and don't fill you up, so you will want to eat a lot. Check the portion size on that fat-free pastry. Are you really going to stop after you've eaten a one-inch-square piece? Most people don't have that much will power. Extra calories are converted to fat, even if the food is made with fat substitutes.

Fat-free salad dressings and mayonnaise are fine because you use small amounts and they encourage you to eat more high-fiber salads and vegetables.

Will soybeans lower cholesterol?

Soybeans are a high-fat food. If you substitute soybeans for meat or chicken, you will lower cholesterol a little bit because you're substituting an unsaturated fat from plants for saturated fat from animals. This reduces cholesterol in two ways: plant protein helps decrease fat absorption and it helps the liver clear cholesterol from the bloodstream more rapidly. However, if you add a lot of soybeans to your diet, you will raise cholesterol because you are eating extra calories. If you want to lower your cholesterol significantly, you need to reduce fat from all sources.

Is bread permitted on a low-fat diet?

Breads that have less than 1 gram of fat per slice are permissible on a low-fat diet, provided that you don't eat more than a couple of slices. Read the labels carefully because all of the following are sold with and without fat: French bread, sourdough bread, pita bread, English muffins, bagels and matzo. Fats add flavor and color and help breads retain moisture and prolong shelf-life. Low-fat breads dry out, become stale very quickly and have a very short shelf-life. They should be stored in the refrigerator or freezer. You can often revive stale bread by sprinkling a little water on the crust and toasting it for a few minutes in the oven.

You should limit even fat-free breads because they are low in fiber, and you can eat a lot of extra calories without feeling full. Whole-grain breads have a little more fiber than "white" breads, but they are still low-fiber foods. Most breads that are labeled "whole wheat" or "rye" are actually made with a high percentage of refined flour. The very dark breads are the only ones that don't have much refined flour, and they usually have fat added to make them moist.

What are the benefits of eating bran?

A high-fat diet increases a woman's chances of developing breast cancer and anyone's chances of having a heart attack. Bran or any other source of fiber helps lower fat absorption. However, eating oat bran does not prevent heart attacks, and eating wheat bran does not prevent breast cancer. Bran has no special benefits over other whole grains, fruits, vegetables and beans that are good sources of fiber.

I read that you can eat meat on a low-fat diet. Why do you recommend restricting meat?

If you want to lower cholesterol or lose weight by changing your diet without taking drugs, your goal is to restrict fat to fewer than 20 grams per day. Three ounces of cooked beef contain 13 grams of fat and no plant fiber. Such a small portion contains more than half of your daily allotment, yet will still leave you hungry.

What about lean beef?

There is no advantage to buying lean beef (20% fat) over regular beef (30% fat). After cooking, they have virtually the same fat and cholesterol content. Rinsing meat in water several times after cooking does reduce the fat content a little, but who wants washed meat? I recommend that you cut out all kinds of meat and eat fish or shellfish only three to four times a week.

Everyone else says chicken and turkey are fine on a low-fat diet.

Even if the skin and fat are removed, the meat of chicken still contains a significant amount of fat and almost no carbohydrate or fiber. One cup of dark meat with the skin and fat removed contains 14 grams of fat. One cup of light meat contains 7 grams of fat, or one-third of your daily 20-gram allotment. And 33 percent of the fat is saturated. It won't hurt if you eat chicken or turkey occasionally. Remember, you can eat whatever you want once or twice a week. But people who eat chicken or turkey every day for lunch or dinner are getting too much fat.

I heard that shellfish are high in cholesterol and should be avoided.

Early studies showed that shellfish were high in cholesterol, but they reported a chemical analysis that measured all of the sterols, including dihydrocholesterol, which does not raise blood cholesterol levels. Newer techniques have shown that shellfish contain far less cholesterol than we originally thought. Shellfish are low in fat and are good sources of protein. You can certainly include them on your list of seafood choices to enjoy three to four times a week.

Is it OK to use prepared spaghetti sauces?

Check the label of your favorite brand. Most of the spaghetti sauces that come in jars are loaded with fat. On the other hand, most of the canned tomato sauces are fat free. You can add mushrooms, chopped onions or green peppers and seasonings such as oregano, thyme and cayenne to add flavor and texture.

Do you recommend the juicers that are advertised so much on TV?

Don't believe the claims you hear on the juicer infomercials. Juice is no more healthful than the fruit or vegetable it was extracted from. Most juicers remove fiber, and most Americans eat only 11 grams of fiber a day when they should be getting 35 grams. A whole orange is full of fiber, so it helps satisfy your hunger with only 65 calories. An 8-ounce glass of orange juice contains 110 calories and doesn't fill you up because it has only a little of the fiber of a whole orange. There is no evidence to support the claim that fiber prevents your body from absorbing minerals and vitamins. In addition to helping you lose weight and control cholesterol, fiber helps prevent constipation, gall bladder disease and colon cancer.

Should I take iron supplements?

A diet rich in iron and fat increases your risk of heart attacks.[44] Iron and copper convert LDL cholesterol to oxidized LDL cholesterol, which forms plaques in arteries. You can find out your iron levels by asking your doctor to check blood iron, iron binding capacity and ferritin. Since blood iron levels vary considerably, they are not a good measure of iron. Ferritin is the form of iron that is stored in your liver, spleen, bone marrow and other tissues. High ferritin levels may show that you have too much iron, but ferritin can be falsely elevated when you have arthritis or other diseases that cause swelling.

You should consider taking iron supplements only if these tests show that you are truly deficient. If you have too much iron, cut back on meat, eggs and other rich sources. You can also donate blood periodically.

Are natural vitamin pills more effective than regular vitamins?

There is no evidence that healthy people need to take vitamin pills, but if you want to take them, don't be taken in by useless claims. The word "natural" on the vitamin label has no meaning. All vitamins are chemically the same, whether they are extracted from rose hips or are manufactured in a chemistry laboratory.

Starch-free, sugar-free, yeast-free and preservative-free vitamins offer no advantage because starch, sugar, yeast and approved preservatives are safe and are found frequently in the foods that you eat. Starch and sugar help to mask the unpleasant taste of some vitamins. Vitamins that are extracted from yeast are perfectly safe, and preservatives help to keep vitamins from breaking down.

It is ridiculous to pay extra for a vitamin C nasal spray because everyone can absorb vitamin C from the intestines. There is no advantage to "timed-release" vitamins because all vitamins are absorbed through your intestines. It doesn't matter whether the vitamin is absorbed in the first few feet of the intestines or the last few feet. However, large doses of niacin can make you itch, so timed-release pills can slow absorption and help to prevent itching.

Do vitamin pills prevent cancer?

Some promoters of vitamins conduct campaigns to convince people that their supplements prevent cancer. They cite a study which shows that

Chinese peasants who take vitamin supplements have lower cancer rates. The Chinese peasants eat a diet that lacks basic nutrients. Giving these people vitamin pills helps to treat the vitamin deficiencies that may increase their chances of developing cancer. However, the American diet is not vitamin deficient and there is no evidence that giving vitamin pills to people who are not nutritionally deficient prevents cancer. The National Cancer Institute, which sponsored the second study, *does not* recommend that Americans take vitamin or mineral supplements. They recommend eating a low-fat, high-fiber diet that is loaded with fruits and vegetables.

Will I get enough vitamin D on a low-fat diet?

Vitamin D is necessary to keep bones strong. Lack of vitamin D also may increase your chances of developing cancer of the prostate and breast cancer. Most of us do not meet our requirements for vitamin D through the foods that we eat. Exposing a couple of inches of skin to sunlight for ten minutes a day provides all the vitamin D we need.

Vitamin D is found in fish, eggs, liver, vitamin D–fortified milk and butter. You can meet your daily needs for vitamin D on a low-fat diet by getting a little sunlight, drinking vitamin D–fortified skim milk and eating fish. If you are a strict vegetarian and stay out of the sun, you should take a supplement with 400 international units of vitamin D.

Should I take fiber supplements?

Several manufacturers claim that fiber supplements will lower cholesterol and prevent heart attacks. You don't need their supplements. You can get all the fiber you need from the foods that you eat. On a low-fat diet you will eat lots of fruits, vegetables, whole grains and beans — all loaded with fiber.

Exercise Questions

What kind of exercise program do you recommend?

What do you want from your exercise program? The goals you set for yourself determine how you should exercise. *If you want to become fit,* you should exercise vigorously enough to raise your pulse at least 20 more beats a minute above resting and hold that rate for at least ten minutes every other day. You can run, walk, skate, cycle, dance, swim, cross-country ski, row or conduct an orchestra. *If you want to lose weight,* try to exercise intensely for at least ten minutes every other day. You will raise your body temperature and keep on burning extra calories even after you have stopped exercising. Swimming is not as good for weight loss as exercise on the ground because water conducts heat away from your body so your metabolism does not stay elevated.

If you want to become a better athlete, you need to train specifically for your sport. *If you want to develop large, strong muscles*, you need to exercise against resistance in successive bouts of not more than fifty consecutive seconds. Usually, that means lifting and lowering a heavy weight three to twelve times in a row for several different exercises. *If you want to become more flexible*, you need a daily program of stretching slowly and deliberately. *If you want to develop coordination* that is necessary to hit a baseball or tennis ball, or to throw a basketball through a hoop, you need to practice these skills over and over again many times a day. *If you want to increase your endurance*, go as hard as you can in short bursts at least once a week, and take one long workout in your sport each week, exercising continuously for at least an hour.

I'm 55 and want to start exercising. If I'm going to buy only one piece of exercise equipment, what should I get?

Virtually everyone over 50 who hasn't exercised in a while should be using a recumbent stationary bicycle. Whatever your age, try a recumbent model before you buy a standard stationary bicycle — or any other piece of exercise equipment. You sit in a contoured chair and pedal with your feet horizontal to your pelvis. Pedal at a comfortable speed, with the bicycle set at the lowest resistance, until your legs feel heavy or until they hurt. Do this every other day until you can pedal for ten to twenty minutes. You can then increase your workout by pedaling faster or increasing the resistance.

Should I exercise every day?

Nobody can exercise vigorously every day. If you think that you can, expect to be injured. All athletic training is done by stressing and recovering. It's called the "hard-easy principle." On one day, you exercise vigorously and your muscles feel sore. Then, for the next few workouts you exercise far less intensely until the soreness disappears. Only then should you attempt another hard workout.

If you do not compete in sports, it is better to exercise only every other day or to alternate sports that stress different parts of your body. For example, on one day, you could stress your legs by running or dancing. On the next day, you could stress your back and shoulders by pulling on a rowing machine. The hard-easy principle applies to your skeletal muscles, not your heart. You can exercise hard on consecutive days as long as you do not use the same set of skeletal muscles. It's much better to exercise vigorously one day and take the next day off than to just lollygag along every day.

I want to start exercising, but I'm afraid of getting injured.

There's a set sequence of symptoms during exercise that precedes injuries. First your legs or arms feel heavy, then they feel sore, then you feel pain in a single spot, and finally that spot hurts all the time, even when you are not moving.

Young people can exercise through the heavy and burning feelings but should stop when they feel pain in a single spot. They can then exercise at a very leisurely pace on the next day. However, when older people exercise through the burning feeling, they should take the next day off or they are very likely to injure themselves.

If you haven't exercised in a long time, exercise up to the point at which your muscles start to burn, and then stop. If you stop immediately when your muscles start to feel heavy and burn, you won't exercise very intensely or very long and you won't become very fit. You can get around this by combining two or more activities in each exercise session. Pick two or more sports that stress different muscle groups; for example, pulling on a rowing machine and jogging. Start out by pulling on the rowing machine until the muscles in your arms or back start to feel sore, and stop. Then go out and run until your leg muscles start to feel sore, and stop. If you do not feel sore on the next day, you can repeat the workout.

How long should I warm up before exercising?

Always start off each workout slowly. Starting off fast increases your chances of injuring yourself. When muscles are stressed before they have a chance to warm up, they are tight and inflexible and at increased risk of tearing. Warming up also increases the force that can be exerted by muscles.

When you exercise, your muscles burn fat and sugar for energy. Less than 30 percent of the energy is used to power your muscles, and more than 70 percent of the energy is lost as heat. So muscle temperature rises whenever you exercise. Resting muscle temperature is around 98 degrees. After you jog slowly for just a few minutes, your muscle temperature can be as high as 101 degrees.

To prevent injury, you need to warm up for only one to three minutes. To develop maximum power, you need to warm up until you start to sweat and your body temperature rises 1 to 2 degrees. The best way to warm up for running is to run slowly, and the best way to warm up for swimming is to swim slowly.

Does stretching before exercising prevent injuries?

There is no evidence that stretching prevents injuries. You are likely to injure yourself if you stretch when your muscles are cold or tired. The older you are, the greater your chances of injury when you stretch. A well-supervised program of stretching can increase flexibility, but you should only stretch *after* your muscles are thoroughly warmed up.

Why is cooling down important?

If you stop exercising suddenly, you can get dizzy, and if you have a weak heart, it may start beating irregularly. Cooling down just means slowing down gradually, and you only have to do it for a few minutes. During exercise, your leg muscles serve as a second heart to help pump blood through your body. When your leg muscles relax, the nearby veins fill up with blood. When the muscles contract, they squeeze the veins, pushing the blood back toward the heart. If you exercise vigorously and stop suddenly, your leg muscles stop contracting and blood can pool in your legs. Your heart may not be able to pump enough blood to your brain to meet its needs, and you will feel dizzy. You may even pass out. Slowing down gradually lets your heart pick up the extra work when your legs stop pumping.

Is it true that you burn the same number of calories by walking or running the same distance?

It depends on how fast you walk. When you run, you burn about 100 calories a mile, no matter how fast you go. You keep the same form at any speed. When you walk slowly, at 3 miles an hour, you burn 64 calories a mile. When you walk fast, at 5 miles an hour, you burn about 128 calories a mile. The faster you walk, the more energy you use with the exaggerated side-to-side motion. Fast walking can be even more vigorous than running, and you are less likely to be injured.

My exercise instructor talks a lot about maximum heart rate. Why is it important?

Virtually every student in an exercise class learns that the fastest rate your heart should beat is determined by the formula 220 minus your age. But that formula applies only to out-of-shape older people. According to the formula, if you are 40 years old, the fastest your heart can beat is 220 minus 40, or 180. If you are 20 years old, the fastest your heart can beat is 220 minus 20, or 200 beats a minute. However, very fit older athletes can have the same maximum heart rates as younger people.

The formula depends only on how strong your skeletal muscles are. Older people who have strong skeletal muscles can have very fast maximum heart rates. Your heart rate is driven by how hard you exercise your muscles. When you start to exercise, your muscles alternately contract and relax. With each contraction, the muscles squeeze blood out of the veins near them. When the muscles relax, the veins near them fill up with blood. So exercise causes your muscles to pump far more blood to your heart. The heart responds to the increased return of blood by beating with more force at a faster rate. The reason that maximum heart rate decreases with aging is that your skeletal muscles weaken and can't drive your heart as hard as when you were younger.

So if you're fit, forget about the formula that the fastest your heart can beat during exercise is 220 minus your age. To make your heart beat faster, all you have to do is make your skeletal muscles stronger.

What is the difference between the exercise pulse rate of a fit person and a sedentary person of the same age?

An out-of-shape person and an in-shape person can both exercise at the same heart rate, but the fit person will move much faster. The more fit you are, the more blood your heart will pump with each beat. So a marathon runner and a novice may both exercise at 140 beats per minute as they run around a track, but the marathon runner will go a lot faster.

Health Questions

Should I be taking aspirin to prevent heart attacks?

Americans take more than 6 billion aspirin tablets each year because they believe they are preventing heart attacks. There are two components to a heart attack: first, over many years, fatty plaques accumulate in arteries and slow blood flow to a trickle. Then a clot forms in the artery to obstruct blood flow completely and cause a heart attack. Aspirin does not stop the formation of plaques; it helps to prevent clots. So aspirin prevents heart attacks only in people who already have significant plaques in their arteries.

Far more important than preventing clotting is preventing the buildup of plaques or reversing plaques that are already in your arteries. You do that with a low-fat diet and lots of fiber. One baby aspirin every other day gives you maximal protection against clotting. Taking doses higher than that does not benefit you further and can cause other side effects, such as stomach upset and bleeding.

My cholesterol is 230. Should I be on a low-fat diet?

Forget about total cholesterol. To judge if your cholesterol is elevated, your doctor should use the relationship of HDL (Healthy) to LDL (Lousy) cholesterol. For every rise in LDL, you need a protective rise in HDL. For example, if your LDL is 90, you need an HDL of at least 35. The chart on page 22 will help you understand the numbers you get from your doctor. If your LDL is over 140, you should be on a low-fat diet regardless of your HDL level.

I'm not terribly overweight, but I have a beer belly. My doctor says that increases my risk of a heart attack. What can I do?

Men who deposit fat primarily in their bellies are far more likely to suffer from heart attacks than men who deposit fat primarily in their hips. The same applies to women. Right now you should be on a low-fat diet, but in the future you may also use a testosterone skin patch. A new study in the *International Journal of Obesity* shows that the male hormone may help to prevent heart attacks in older men, as long as it is not taken by mouth. Testosterone taken by mouth goes to the liver and decreases production of the good HDL cholesterol. When taken by patch, testosterone does not go to the liver and does not reduce HDL.

Men go into a change similar to menopause, even though the change may be more gradual in women. A man's blood levels of testosterone drop more than 40 percent from age 50 to 70. What happens to men with fat bellies who are given testosterone by skin patch? Only good things. It reduces their belly fat and lowers cholesterol, blood pressure and blood sugar. Having a lot of belly fat causes dietary fat to be shunted to the liver, which converts it to cholesterol that forms fatty plaques that plug up arteries. Replacing testosterone with a patch reduces body fat and increases muscle. With less belly fat, less dietary fat is shunted to the liver to be converted to cholesterol, so blood levels of cholesterol drop.

Do I really need to worry more about having a heart attack because I'm bald?

An article in the *Journal of the American Medical Association* reported that baldness on the top of the head is associated with an increased risk of having a heart attack. This study does not show that most bald men will get heart attacks. It only demonstrates a weak association between top-of-the-head baldness and heart attacks. It is far weaker than the association of heart attacks with smoking, high blood pressure, elevated blood levels of cholesterol and triglycerides, storing fat in your belly, or having xanthomas (yellow spots on your upper eyelids).

Hormones may explain the association between baldness and heart attacks. The male hormone, testosterone, is necessary for potency. A derivative of testosterone called dihydrotestosterone causes top-of-the-head baldness and also lowers the good HDL cholesterol that prevents heart attacks.

Is it possible to have a cholesterol that's too low?

Lowering your cholesterol reduces your chances of developing a heart attack. Several reports claim that low cholesterol is associated with an increased risk of developing lung cancer, alcoholism, depression, suicide and accidents. None of the studies show that low cholesterol causes these conditions. It's the other way around. People with many chronic diseases have poor appetites and eat less, so their cholesterol levels go down.

How soon will my cholesterol level go down if I go on a low-fat diet?

All cholesterol changes that you will get from a change in your diet will occur within ten days after you make the change. If you still do not have a proper ratio of LDL to HDL after ten days, you need to make additional changes in your diet or begin medication. Most people can achieve a satisfactory cholesterol ratio with stringent fat restriction alone.

I'm very worried about osteoporosis. What can I do to prevent it?

A woman's bones are strongest when she is 20 years old. Each year after that, she loses a bit more calcium, and her bones become a little weaker. At the menopause, her yearly bone loss triples, and she continues to lose bone at a high rate for several years. This process is so relentless that it will eventually cause every woman to develop osteoporosis if she lives long enough.

Some women are at increased risk of developing osteoporosis, including those who go into the menopause before the average age of 52 and those who are very skinny or have a family history of osteoporosis. Other factors that increase a woman's chances of developing osteoporosis are drinking, smoking, eating a diet low in calcium, not exercising and having a pale complexion.

Most doctors give women estrogen at the menopause. However, estrogen does not replace bone. It only slows down the rate at which bone is lost. Two drugs, etidronate and calcitonin, can be used to make bones denser and stronger after the menopause.

What can I do about a stomach ulcer?

Eighty percent of stomach and intestinal ulcers can be cured by taking antibiotics for one or two weeks. Americans spend millions of dollars each year for medications like ranitidine (Zantac) or omeprazole (Prilosec) to treat ulcers. These drugs decrease stomach acidity, but, unlike antibiotics, they do not cure ulcers.

If you have stomach or chest pain that increases when you are hungry and lessens immediately after you eat, belching, burping, a sour taste in your mouth or a white-coated tongue, your doctor should order an x-ray to rule out a cancer and check for an ulcer, and you should get a blood test to see if you are infected with a bacterium called *Helicobacter pylori*.[45] If the blood test shows infection, you can be cured by taking metronidazole, 250 mg four times a day for one week; amoxicillin, 250 mg four times a day for one week; and omeprazole, 10 mg once a day for one week. Then repeat the blood test twelve weeks after you finish treatment. If the *Helicobacter* test is still high, you may need a second course of antibiotics.

If you have an acidic stomach and are not infected with *Helicobacter*, you should avoid coffee, tea, chocolate and any drinks with bubbles and may have to take medication to protect your stomach for the rest of your life.

CHAPTER 13

275 Truly Low-Fat, Truly Delicious Recipes

My recipes **don't use any oil, margarine or butter**. Most "low-fat" cookbooks and diet plans ask you to reduce the amount of oil you use. They call for a tablespoon of fat where a traditional recipe used half a cup. This sounds good, but in practice, most cooks don't measure. You pour in a little puddle of oil that looks like about a tablespoon. In reality, it may be two or three. Then if the food absorbs the oil and begins to stick to the pan, you add a little more.

I know that if I have oil in my kitchen, I will use it. So my recipes don't call for any cooking fats at all. For the same reason, you won't find even small quantities of other high-fat ingredients in the recipes. **No cheese, no nuts, no meat (including chicken), no eggs**. Egg whites have no fat, but can you really trust yourself to throw those high-fat yolks down the drain? I can't. **Keep temptation out of your kitchen!**

Symbols

The symbols next to the recipes help you identify some special features at a glance.

  Quick and Easy. These recipes take little preparation and cook quickly. They are ideal when you are in a hurry or don't want much fuss. If you've never done much cooking, start with a few of the Quick and Easy recipes. Please note: **None of my recipes are hard or tricky!** Some just have longer cooking times or take a little more time to prepare lots of ingredients.

Freezes Well. You can prepare a large quantity of these recipes and freeze the surplus for future meals. That's how you can build your own supply of "fast food" that just needs to be reheated in your microwave.

Master Recipe. This symbol marks recipes with basic techniques or favorite seasonings that can be used over and over with various combinations of vegetables, beans, fruits or grains.

Low-Fat/Low-Fiber. These symbols call your attention to recipes that include seafood, dairy products, sweets or refined grains. You will need to limit your portion sizes of those ingredients (see Serving Sizes, below).

Unusual Ingredient. Some of my recipes include ingredients that may not be familiar to you. The Glossary of Unusual Ingredients (page 314) explains them and tells where you may be able to find them.

Serving Sizes

To help you plan your meals, an estimated number of servings is given with each recipe. Serving sizes are generally based on 1- to 2-cup portions for main dishes and ½- to 1-cup portions for side dishes and desserts. No serving numbers are given for snacks, spice mixes, condiments, sauces and other recipes that are not major parts of a meal.

I want to emphasize that the number of servings listed with a recipe is not meant to dictate how much you can eat. **You can eat as much as you like of the recipes made with fruits, vegetables, whole grains and beans** to feel comfortably full. Portion sizes of low-fat/low-fiber foods should be limited (see Table 7 on page 77); recipes that use these ingredients are clearly marked with the ▣ ▣ ▣ ▣ symbols. You need only limit the amount of the specific low-fat/low-fiber ingredient. For example, if you are serving Couscous with Seven Vegetables (page 148), put ½ **cup** of couscous in your bowl and top it with as much of the vegetable stew as you like.

You *won't* find the usual listing of calories and food components with my recipes. That's because trying to count calories sets you up for failure. If you're still looking for calorie counts on recipes or food labels, reread the section on why counting calories doesn't work (page 33).

I do ask you to count grams of fat, but only in foods that are not in your basic 15 grams each day (see page 74). *Everything you make from my recipes counts as part of your basic 15 grams.* The only ingredients in my recipes that may contain more than 1 gram of fat per serving are the beans and seafood, and these foods are your essential sources of protein. The beans and seafood listed in these recipes contain no more than 3 grams of fat per serving. They are counted in your basic 15 grams.

Poetic License

My recipes are meant to inspire you and help you learn to make low-fat food taste delicious. They are not rigid formulae. If there is a vegetable or other ingredient you don't like, leave it out or substitute something else. The recipes marked with the "master recipe" symbol ⚄ are especially good for swapping ingredients and experimenting with new combinations.

Most cooks use "a handful of this and a pinch of that" instead of measuring precisely. Low-fat cooking doesn't have any fussy ingredients that make recipes fail, so feel free to improvise. If you want to add a little more or less of something than the recipe calls for, go right ahead.

To Peel or Not to Peel?

Vegetable and fruit skins are loaded with fiber and nutrients. You don't want to throw them away unless you have to. Recipes in lots of other cookbooks tell you to peel potatoes, apples, eggplants and everything else, whether you need to or not.

If the skin is bitter or very tough, it probably needs to be removed. But many vegetables that most people peel have completely edible skins. Potatoes and carrots just need to be scrubbed; peeling is time-consuming and wasteful. Apple and pear skins add color and crunch. Cucumbers (unwaxed) look pretty in a salad if you score the skin with a fork before slicing instead of peeling.

When I make casseroles with eggplants, tomatoes and other vegetables that are usually peeled, I try them once with the skins left on to see if it makes an objectionable difference. Usually they're just fine, and I can save time while adding fiber.

If you decide to peel, you may be able to find other uses for the discards. Orange skins can be made into marmalade or candied peel. Most vegetable scraps can be added to stock.

If you think peeling is important for the texture or appearance of your dish, go ahead, but at least think about it before you automatically throw away valuable fiber and vitamins.

You don't have to worry about lumpy gravy, curdled sauces or fallen soufflés because you didn't follow the directions exactly. **Low-fat cooking is easy!**

Do remember that spices cooked in water develop less flavor than those cooked in fat. If you are accustomed to cooking spices in oil, you may find that you need more of your favorite spices to get a similar flavor. If the quantity of a spice in one of my recipes seems alarmingly large, start out with a smaller amount, and taste as you go.

Main Dishes of Vegetables, Grains and Beans

These main-dish recipes are the staples of a low-fat diet. They are high in fiber, contain no added fat and are easy to prepare. All that is needed to complete a meal is a salad and perhaps some bread. They are easy to make in large quantities and most will freeze well. You can make up a pot on the weekend and have ready-to-serve meals for busy weeknights.

Many of these dishes make delicious sandwich fillings. For a quick lunch, heat a small portion in the microwave and stuff it into a pita bread with some lettuce and perhaps tomato or cucumber slices.

You can always adjust the ingredients and the quantities in my recipes to suit your own taste. Make substitutions to use what you have on hand or what looks good in the produce department. If you don't like a particular vegetable, leave it out. Adjust the spices and seasonings as you wish, tasting as you go. But be adventurous! Use these recipes for inspiration, and invent your own combinations. It's hard to go wrong.

My Famous Bean-Eggplant-Tomato Casserole

I make a huge quantity — 3 or 4 times the recipe — and freeze it in individual meal-size containers. Serve it with a green salad for supper or stuff it into a pita bread for lunch.

> 1 pound dried kidney beans or 15-bean soup mix
> 2 onions, chopped
> 4 cloves garlic, minced
> 2 green peppers, chopped
> 3 cans (28 ounces each) plum tomatoes, chopped
> 2 tablespoons fresh oregano or 2 teaspoons dried
> 1 tablespoon fresh thyme or 1 teaspoon dried
> 2 bay leaves
> 1/4 teaspoon cayenne or to taste
> 2 eggplants

Soak the beans overnight. Drain the beans and cover them with water in a large pot; bring to a boil and cook until the beans are tender, 1 to 2 hours. Drain off any excess liquid. Meanwhile, in a second pot, bring the onion, garlic, green pepper, tomatoes, and the seasonings to a boil and simmer for 10 minutes. Dice the eggplant and add it to the pot. (You can peel the eggplant if you wish; I never do.) Stir in the cooked beans and simmer 20 minutes.

10 to 12 servings

Mexican Vegetable Stew

This dish is as colorful as the Mexican flag if you cook the green beans and squash until they're just crisp-tender.

> 2 onions, sliced
> 1 sweet red pepper, cut in strips
> 1 green pepper, cut in strips
> 2 cloves garlic, minced
> 1 1/2 cups bouillon (see page 187)
> 1 teaspoon cumin
> 1 tablespoon fresh oregano or 1 teaspoon dried
> 1/2 teaspoon fennel seeds
> 1/4 teaspoon red pepper flakes or to taste
> 2 red potatoes, diced

1 sweet potato, diced
2 cups green beans, cut in 1-inch pieces
1 zucchini, sliced
1 yellow squash, sliced
1 can chick peas, undrained, or 2 cups cooked
2 ears corn cut in 1-inch pieces or 1 cup corn kernels
2 tablespoons lime juice
½ cup cilantro or Italian parsley leaves, chopped

Bring the onion, red and green peppers, garlic and ½ cup bouillon to a boil in a large pot and simmer 5 minutes. Stir in the spices, red potato and sweet potato; cover and simmer 10 minutes, adding more bouillon if needed. Add the beans; cook 5 minutes more. Stir in the remaining bouillon and bring to a boil. Add the zucchini and yellow squash, chick peas, corn and lime juice. Reduce the heat and simmer 5 minutes, or until all the vegetables are tender. Garnish with cilantro or parsley.

10 to 12 servings

Vegetarian Chili I

Chili is right up there with my vegetable curries at the top of my list of favorite dishes. Fat-free vegetarian chilies come in many forms, and I hope you will feel free to improvise on the recipes in this chapter. You can use different kinds of beans; you can cook the beans from scratch or use canned ones; and you can add just spices or combine the beans with a whole host of vegetables. This recipe starts with dried beans, but it is just as tasty using canned red kidney beans.

1 pound small red chili beans
4 cups bouillon or more as needed (see page 187)
1 large onion, chopped
2 cloves garlic, minced
2 stalks celery, chopped
1 green pepper, chopped
2 dried red peppers, crushed, or ¼ teaspoon cayenne pepper or to taste
4 tablespoons chili powder
1 teaspoon oregano
1 teaspoon cumin
1 can (28 ounces) plum tomatoes, chopped
1 cup bulgur
1 cup frozen corn
2 tablespoons Worcestershire sauce
Cilantro, chopped

Soak the beans overnight; drain and rinse. In a large pot, cover the beans with bouillon and bring to a boil; simmer gently while chopping the vegetables. Add the onion, garlic, celery, green pepper and spices and simmer until the beans are soft, about 40 to 60 minutes. Add the tomatoes with their juice and the bulgur; simmer another 20 minutes. Add the

A Pepper Primer

Peppers come in hundreds of varieties, ranging from the familiar green (bell) pepper to the exotic shapes and fiery tastes of Thai chiles and Scotch bonnet peppers. Here's a brief guide to the peppers I use in my recipes and some others you may want to try.

Warning! Always wear rubber gloves when preparing fresh or dried hot peppers!

Sweet fresh peppers: Green peppers are a low-fat kitchen staple for casseroles, soups and salads. Red and yellow bell peppers taste almost the same, perhaps a bit sweeter. They are usually more expensive, but their pretty colors make them worthwhile. Other mild peppers include Italian frying peppers, cubanelle peppers and banana peppers. They are usually a lighter green, thinner and longer than bell peppers. You can't always tell whether a pepper is sweet or hot by its appearance; if in doubt, ask your grocer.

Hot fresh peppers: Jalapeños are cone-shaped, about two inches long and dark green (sometimes red); two or three will add plenty of heat to a whole pot. The fieriest chiles are small and dark green or red; add one or two, slivered, to your recipe and taste before adding more. The larger fresh chiles, such as New Mexico or Anaheim, are usually fairly mild when cooked, but they have enough heat so you'll want to be careful handling them while raw (wear gloves) and remove the seeds, which can be very hot even in the sweeter chiles.

To roast fresh peppers or chiles: Roasted bell peppers are delicious in salads or as a side dish. Remove the stem and seeds, slice lengthwise or crossways into ½-inch pieces, spread on a foil-covered cookie sheet and broil about 5 minutes. You can also use this method to roast and peel whole chiles: remove the stems and seeds and arrange the whole chiles in a single layer on a foil-covered cookie sheet. Broil 5 minutes or until the skin is blistered and charred; turn and broil the other side for 5 minutes. Place the chiles in a paper bag, close the top and allow them to cool. Most of the skin will peel off easily; a few remaining bits won't hurt.

corn and Worcestershire sauce and cook 5 minutes more. Ladle into bowls and sprinkle with chopped cilantro. Serve with no-fat tortilla chips.

8 to 10 servings

Hot peppers from the spice shelf: Cayenne or ground red pepper, red pepper flakes and whole dried red pepper pods all provide lots of heat. Add a little at a time and taste as you go. The dried red pepper spices are generally interchangeable in recipes, so use the kind you prefer. A pinch of cayenne (⅛ teaspoon or less) is about equal to ½ teaspoon red pepper flakes or one small pepper pod, crumbled. The amount of heat varies tremendously between brands and with age, so start cautiously when you use a new kind or a fresh batch. It's easy to add more hot pepper to your recipe — and impossible to remove it.

Hot pepper sauces: Tabasco is the best-known of the liquid pepper seasonings, but there are lots of other brands. Because they contain vinegar, they will add a slightly different flavor to your recipe than dried hot peppers. Some have other spices or "secret ingredients" as well. Hot pepper sauces can be used as a cooking ingredient or added at the table. Try a few and pick your favorites.

Dried chiles: If you like Mexican and southwestern cooking, experiment with different kinds of dried chiles, starting with my recipes for Vegetarian Chili on pages 137 and 140. Large supermarkets usually have dried Anaheim chiles, and Hispanic markets carry a bewildering array of varieties — usually without any labels to guide you. As with fresh chiles, the large ones are *usually* milder and the small ones will be hot. To prepare dried chiles for cooking, remove and discard the stems and seeds, and tear the pods into pieces (wear gloves). Soak the pieces in hot water to cover for 15 minutes or more. Put the chiles and a little of their soaking liquid in a blender or food processor; turn the switch on and off until you have a chunky puree. Add a little of the puree to your recipe, cook about 5 minutes, then taste for heat before adding the rest. If you need more liquid in your recipe, use the rest of the soaking water.

Canned and bottled peppers: You can buy mild green chiles, chopped or whole, in small cans in the Hispanic section of most supermarkets; they are interchangeable with roasted fresh green chiles and are quick and easy to use. I'm sometimes able to find large jars of delicious roasted red peppers in the Italian section — for salads or garnishes. Finally, pickled peppers come in all shades of heat and can be used in salads or as condiments.

Vegetarian Chili II

This chili is made with the big, dark red dried peppers that are appearing in more and more supermarkets. If you can't find them, just use 3 to 4 tablespoons of your favorite chili powder. You can use canned beans if you wish.

> 1 pound dried kidney beans or pink beans
> 6 dried Anaheim or New Mexico chiles
> 3 cups boiling water
> 1 cup bulgur
> 1 cup hot bouillon (see page 187)
> 1 onion, chopped
> 2 cloves garlic, minced
> 1 green pepper, chopped
> 1 can (28 ounces) plum tomatoes
> 2 teaspoons ground cumin
> 2 tablespoons fresh oregano or 1 teaspoon dried

Soak the beans overnight; drain and rinse. Add water to cover, bring to a boil again and simmer gently for an hour or more, or until the beans are tender. Drain, reserving the cooking liquid.

Meanwhile, prepare the chiles: Remove the stems and seeds and discard. Tear the pods into pieces, place them in a bowl and cover with boiling water. Soak for 30 minutes. Put chiles and their soaking water in a blender and blend to a smooth puree.

Place the bulgur in a bowl and pour the hot bouillon over it; soak for 15 minutes.

In a second pot, cook the chopped onion, garlic and green pepper in ½ cup of the bean cooking liquid until the vegetables are softened, about 10 minutes. Add the tomatoes and their juice, breaking up the tomatoes. Add the chile puree, cumin and oregano; simmer gently. Add the soaked bulgur to the vegetable mixture. Stir in the cooked beans. Simmer the chili for 30 minutes, stirring occasionally to prevent sticking; add some of the bean liquid as needed if the chili is too thick.

Anaheim chiles vary in heat; if the chili is too mild for your taste, add a little cayenne pepper. Serve the chili with no-fat tortilla chips and a green salad.

8 to 10 servings

Black Beans

This is a good basic recipe for cooking dried black beans, to be used in many ways. Serve them over brown rice, accompanied by a green salad. Fill pita bread with beans, and top with chopped lettuce and tomato. Or puree some of the beans in a blender to make a delicious soup, stirring in a little bouillon to the desired consistency.

> 1 pound dried black beans
> bouillon to cover beans (see page 187)
> 2 onions, chopped
> 1 bay leaf
> 2 cloves garlic, minced
> 1 can (28 ounces) plum tomatoes, chopped
> 1 teaspoon hot pepper sauce or to taste
> 2 teaspoons cumin
> 2 tablespoons chili powder
> 2 carrots, chopped
> 2 stalks celery, chopped
> 1 orange, quartered (unpeeled)
> ½ cup Italian parsley, chopped
> Cooked brown rice (optional)

Soak the beans overnight; drain and rinse. Cover the beans with bouillon in a large pot; bring to a boil and simmer 1 hour. Add the remaining ingredients except the parsley and simmer 1½ hours, or until the beans are tender, adding more water if needed. Remove the bay leaf and orange quarters and serve over brown rice; sprinkle with parsley.

6 to 8 servings

Quick Chili

If you're a fast chopper, you can have this chili ready in 20 minutes. It's great served with salsa, chopped lettuce and fat-free tortilla chips.

1 onion, chopped
2 cloves garlic, minced
1 green pepper, chopped
1 can (28 ounces) plum tomatoes, chopped
2 teaspoons chili powder
2 teaspoons cumin
2 teaspoons paprika
Pinch cayenne or to taste
2 cans kidney beans or black beans, undrained

Combine all the ingredients except the beans in a large pot, bring to a boil and simmer 10 minutes. Stir in the beans and cook 5 minutes more.

4 to 6 servings

Vegetable Curry I

I never get tired of inventing new vegetable curry combinations. Try this recipe, and then use it as the basic formula for your own experiments. You can use virtually any vegetable that looks good in your produce department, as well as frozen vegetables. I serve my vegetable curries on a bed of brown rice, with a spoonful of yogurt and one of chutney on the edge.

1 large onion, chopped
4 stalks celery, chopped
1 green pepper, chopped
1 cup bouillon (see page 187)
1 tablespoon turmeric
1 tablespoon curry powder
1 teaspoon red pepper flakes or to taste
1 can (28 ounces) plum tomatoes, chopped
4 carrots, sliced
2 red potatoes, diced
1 head cauliflower, broken into florets
1 bunch broccoli, stems sliced and head in florets
2 zucchini, diced
1/2 pound mushrooms, sliced

2 cans chick peas, undrained
½ cup raisins
1 cup low-fat yogurt (optional)
Cooked brown rice

Bring the onion, celery, green pepper and bouillon to a boil in a large pot and simmer 10 minutes. Add the spices, tomatoes, carrot and potato and cook about 15 minutes, or until the carrots are barely tender. Add the cauliflower and the broccoli stems; when the stems start to get tender (after about 10 minutes), add the broccoli florets, zucchini, mushrooms, chick peas and raisins. Cook until all the vegetables are crisp-tender, 5 to 10 more minutes. Stir in the yogurt if desired, and serve over brown rice.

6 to 8 servings

Vegetable Curry II

Here's an example of a vegetable curry made with several individual spices. I don't turn up my nose at curry powder, as some purist cooks do, because it's so convenient and I love its flavor. But I also like to try different spices in varying amounts. If you like these combinations, you may want to consult some Indian cookbooks for more ideas.

1 onion, chopped
3 cloves garlic, minced
½ cup bouillon (see page 187)
2 potatoes, diced
1 head cabbage, cut in chunks
1 head cauliflower, in florets
½ pound green beans, cut in 1-inch pieces
2 teaspoons cumin
1 teaspoon ground coriander
1 teaspoon ginger
1 teaspoon turmeric
Pinch cayenne or to taste
1 cup frozen peas, thawed
Cooked brown rice

Bring the onion, garlic and bouillon to a boil in a large pot and simmer 10 minutes. Add the potato, cabbage, cauliflower, beans and spices and cook 30 minutes. Stir in the peas and serve over brown rice.

6 to 8 servings

Cooking Times For Vegetables

When you cook lots of kinds of vegetables together, you want them all to come out crisp and tender, not mushy. But different vegetables take different lengths of time to cook. I find it helpful to group vegetables as long cookers, medium cookers and short cookers. Then I add them to the pot in order, so they all get cooked through and none are overcooked. Old, tough vegetables will take longer than the times given below, while very young and tender ones will cook quickly.

Long-Cooking Vegetables
Cook 15 to 20 minutes or more
Beets
Carrots
Celery
Celery root
Onions
Potatoes
Sweet potatoes
Turnips
Winter squash
Medium-Cooking Vegetables
Cook 5 to 10 minutes
Asparagus
Cabbage
Green beans
Most frozen vegetables
  (check package directions)
Mushrooms
Okra
Peas
Zucchini

Medium-Cooking Vegetables
Cook 10 to 15 minutes
Broccoli
Brussels sprouts
Cauliflower
Eggplant
Fennel
Green peppers
Kale
Kohlrabi
Lima beans
Parsnips
Quick-Cooking Vegetables
Cook less than 5 minutes
Bean sprouts
Corn
Snow Peas
Spinach
Swiss chard

Okra-Potato Curry

I love the gummy texture of sliced okra in gumbo, but some people don't. The whole okra in this curry tastes — and feels — like an entirely different vegetable.

> 2 onions, sliced
> 4 cloves garlic, minced
> 1/2 cup bouillon
> 1 pound small whole okra
> 4 medium potatoes, diced

1 teaspoon ground coriander
1 teaspoon ground cumin
1 teaspoon nutmeg
1 teaspoon mustard
1 teaspoon fenugreek
1 tablespoon grated gingerroot
Cooked brown rice (optional)

Bring the onion, garlic and bouillon to a boil in a large pot and simmer 5 minutes. Add all of the other ingredients and simmer, covered, 20 minutes, or until the potatoes are tender. Serve with brown rice if desired.

4 to 6 servings

Sweet Potato and Parsnip Curry

What an odd-sounding combination! Sometimes you just have to trust me.

2 onions, sliced
6 cloves garlic, minced
2 jalapeño chiles, seeded and minced
1 tablespoon mustard seed
1 tablespoon grated gingerroot
1 tablespoon curry powder
¼ cup bouillon
½ pound sweet potatoes, peeled and chopped
½ pound parsnips, peeled and chopped
1 can (28 ounces) plum tomatoes
Juice of 2 lemons
Cooked brown rice (optional)

Bring the onions, garlic, chilies, spices and bouillon to a boil in a large pot and simmer 5 to 10 minutes. Add the sweet potatoes, parsnips, tomatoes and lemon juice; cover and simmer 15 minutes, or until the vegetables are tender but not mushy. Serve over brown rice if desired.

4 to 6 servings

Lentil-Eggplant Curry

Lentils are a wonderfully versatile legume. They are natural partners with many different spices and herbs and combine well with other vegetables. In this curry, you cook them just long enough so they are tender but still firm.

> 1 cup lentils
> 3 cups bouillon (see page 187)
> 1 teaspoon turmeric
> 1 tablespoon curry powder
> 1 teaspoon red pepper flakes or to taste
> 2 onions, sliced
> 3 stalks celery, chopped
> 1 green pepper, diced
> 2 medium potatoes, diced
> 1 medium eggplant, peeled and diced
> 1 cup nonfat yogurt
> Cooked brown rice

Bring the lentils, bouillon and spices to a boil in a large pot and simmer while cutting up the vegetables. Add the onion, celery and green pepper and simmer 10 minutes. Add the potato and eggplant and cook 20 minutes, or until both the potatoes and the lentils are soft. Stir in the yogurt and serve over brown rice.

6 to 8 servings

Vegetable Biryani

Indian cooks make a biryani by sealing the ingredients in a pot with a flour crust. My version captures the wonderful fragrance and is very easy to prepare, in spite of the long list of ingredients.

> 3 cups bouillon (see page 187)
> 1½ cups brown rice
> ¼ teaspoon saffron
> 1 teaspoon turmeric
> 1 onion, chopped
> 1 small sweet potato, diced
> 1 carrot, diced
> ½ head cauliflower, broken into small florets

1 green pepper, diced
½ cup golden raisins
2 teaspoons grated gingerroot
1 teaspoon cumin
1 teaspoon coriander
½ teaspoon cinnamon
¼ teaspoon cayenne or to taste
1 cup canned or cooked chick peas
½ cup frozen baby peas
1 tomato, diced
¼ cup cilantro leaves, chopped (optional)
Mango chutney (optional)

Bring 2½ cups of the bouillon to a boil in a large pot; add the rice, saffron and turmeric; cover and simmer 30 minutes. Meanwhile, heat the remaining ½ cup of bouillon in a separate pot and simmer the onion, sweet potato, carrot, cauliflower, green pepper, raisins and spices 15 minutes, or until the vegetables are barely tender. Stir the vegetables into the rice, add the chick peas, peas and tomato, and cook, covered, 10 to 15 minutes, or until liquid is absorbed. Garnish with cilantro leaves and serve with chutney, if desired.

6 to 8 servings

Bright Yellow Dal

Dal is a thick puree of spiced lentils or split peas that can be yellow, orange, green or brown depending on the legume you choose. Serve it with a green salad and pita bread, or combine it with other Indian-inspired dishes for a multicourse ethnic feast.

2 cups yellow lentils or split peas
6 cups bouillon (see page 187)
6 cloves garlic, minced
1 teaspoon red pepper flakes or to taste
1 teaspoon turmeric
2 teaspoons cumin
½ cup cilantro, chopped

Bring all the ingredients except the cilantro to a boil in a large pot and simmer, covered, for 45 minutes. Stir frequently during the last half of the cooking time. Remove from the heat and stir briskly with a whisk or large spoon to mash the lentils or split peas into a creamy puree. (You can use a blender if you want a really smooth dal, but I find the hand-mashed version more interesting.) Stir in most of the cilantro and sprinkle a little on top for garnish.

6 to 8 servings

Couscous with Seven Vegetables

The secret of this Moroccan-inspired stew is *harissa*, an indispensable spice mixture for the low-fat cook. If you keep a batch on hand in your refrigerator, you can turn just about any combination of vegetables and beans into an exotic treat. Traditionally, couscous is cooked by steaming it in a special utensil over the stew. The quick method I use yields a tasty, fluffy grain that's so easy you will want to make it often. Try this basic recipe with green peppers, peas, fennel, green beans, mushrooms, pumpkin, parsnips, cabbage, cauliflower, broccoli, eggplant, celery, etc., etc., etc. — no one will complain if you use more than seven vegetables.

> 2 onions, chopped
> 6 carrots, sliced in 1-inch pieces
> 2 turnips, peeled and cubed
> 1 butternut squash, peeled and cubed
> 1 can (28 ounces) plum tomatoes, chopped
> 4 cups bouillon, divided (see page 187)
> ½ teaspoon turmeric
> 1 teaspoon harissa (page 307) or to taste
> 3 cups cooked chick peas, or 2 cans, undrained
> 4 small zucchini, sliced
> ½ cup raisins
> 1 cup couscous

Bring the onion, carrots, turnips, butternut squash, tomatoes, 2 cups of the bouillon and the seasonings to a boil in a large pot. Simmer 30 minutes, or until all the vegetables are tender. Stir in the chick peas, zucchini and raisins and simmer 5 to 10 minutes.

Meanwhile, cook the couscous: 20 minutes before serving, bring the remaining 2 cups of bouillon to a boil. Add the couscous and cook 2 minutes, stirring constantly. Remove from the heat, cover and let stand 15 minutes. Fluff with a fork. Serve the vegetables over the couscous and pass additional harissa — with a warning about its firepower!

6 to 8 servings

Summer Couscous

This is best with vine-ripened tomatoes and fresh artichokes, but you can make it any time of the year by substituting canned plum tomatoes and frozen artichokes.

> 5 cups bouillon, divided (page 187)
> 1 cup couscous
> 2 onions, chopped
> 3 cloves garlic, minced
> 1 sweet red pepper, chopped
> 3 small red potatoes, diced
> ½ teaspoon harissa (page 307) or to taste
> 4 ripe tomatoes, chopped
> 4 cooked artichoke hearts, cut in wedges
> 1 can chick peas, undrained, or 2 cups cooked
> ½ pound spinach, chopped
> ¼ cup Italian parsley, chopped
> ¼ cup lemon juice
> Freshly ground black pepper

Bring 2 cups of the bouillon to a boil in a medium saucepan, add the couscous and cook 2 minutes, stirring constantly. Remove from the heat, cover and let stand 15 minutes.

Meanwhile, place the onion, garlic and red pepper in ½ cup of the bouillon in a large pot; bring to a boil and simmer 10 minutes. Add the remaining 2½ cups of bouillon, potato and harissa and simmer 15 minutes. Add the tomatoes, artichoke hearts, chick peas and spinach and cook an additional 5 minutes, or until the spinach is wilted. Stir in the parsley and lemon juice. Fluff the couscous with a fork and divide it into serving bowls. Spoon the vegetables over the couscous and serve with ground pepper and additional harissa to taste.

4 to 6 servings

Ethiopian Lentils

I like these spicy lentils with brown rice and sliced tomatoes or a green salad. They make a wonderful stuffing for pita bread, too.

> 1 pound lentils
> 6 cups bouillon (see page 187)
> 6 mild green chiles, roasted, peeled, seeded and chopped (see page 138) or
>   1 bell pepper, chopped, and 1 can (4 ounces) green chiles, chopped
> 2 red onions, chopped
> 2 cloves garlic, minced
> 2 tablespoons Berbere spice mix (page 307)

Canned Tomato Choices

I usually prefer fresh or frozen vegetables for cooking but tomatoes are the exception. Canned tomatoes work just fine in almost any cooked recipe. I cook with fresh tomatoes only when I have a bumper crop from my garden. Supermarkets carry dozens of kinds and sizes of canned tomatoes that are convenient and delicious. My recipes usually call for canned plum tomatoes or tomato sauce because those are my favorites. I'm sure some of the other types would work just as well, so feel free to experiment. Here's what I found on a recent shopping trip:

Tomato sauce: 8-ounce, 15-ounce or 29-ounce cans. Tomato sauce is smooth and not too thick, with a little bit of seasoning herbs and spices. I buy the large cans and keep my pantry well stocked, since I use so much. Recipes made with tomato sauce usually freeze well, so I always cook enough for leftovers.

Whole plum tomatoes: 14.5-ounce or 28-ounce cans (sometimes labeled Italian-style). For recipes that use whole tomatoes, I like these best because they're meaty and have lots of flavor. To chop them, cut them in pieces with a knife while they're still in the can or break them up with a spoon after you pour them into your cooking pot. As with tomato sauce, I always buy the largest size.

Whole tomatoes: 14.5-ounce or 28-ounce cans. These are the plain round tomatoes. I find them more watery and less flavorful than plum tomatoes, but you can use them interchangeably.

Crushed tomatoes: 28-ounce cans. This mixture of broken-up plum tomatoes and tomato puree makes an acceptable substitute for whole plum tomatoes but you may need to add a little liquid.

Freshly ground black pepper
Yogurt (optional)

Bring the lentils and bouillon to a boil in a large pot and simmer 10 minutes. Add the chiles, onion, garlic and spice mix and cook, covered, over low heat 30 minutes, or until most of the liquid is absorbed. Serve with ground black pepper to taste and a dollop of yogurt, if desired.

6 to 8 servings

Tomato puree: 10.75-ounce or 29-ounce cans. Smooth and a little thicker than tomato sauce, without added seasoning. I find the flavor slightly sweeter and less interesting.

Tomato paste: 6-ounce or 18-ounce cans. Tomato paste is very thick with a strong, concentrated flavor. It cannot be substituted directly for any of the other types of tomatoes. If it's all you have on hand, dilute it with stock or water.

Stewed tomatoes: 14.5-ounce cans. Here, tomatoes are cooked with bits of onion, celery and peppers, and various seasonings. Several new varieties are available with ethnic themes such as "salsa" or "Italian-style." I haven't tried them yet since I like to make my own combinations.

Other Tomato Products

Bottled spaghetti sauces: A few fat-free varieties are being offered, but most of these are high-fat foods. Read the labels carefully.

Tomato juice and tomato cocktail mixes: Great for drinking and as a cooking liquid.

Tomato aspic: Jelled tomato juice with seasonings and sugar added; for salads, not for cooking.

Sun-dried tomatoes: I'm still experimenting with these as a cooking ingredient and in salads, but so far I'm not convinced they're worth their high price. Avoid the ones that are packed in oil.

Spicy Chick Peas and Spinach

Chick peas are my very favorite beans. If you have any leftovers, this combination makes a tasty salad, too.

>   1 large onion, chopped
>   4 cloves garlic, minced
>   6 carrots, sliced thin
>   1 cup bouillon (see page 187)
>   ½ teaspoon harissa (page 307)
>   1 pound chick peas, cooked, or 3 cans, undrained
>   ¼ cup fresh cilantro, chopped
>   1 pound fresh spinach, rinsed and torn in pieces
>   Cooked brown rice or couscous

Bring the onion, garlic, carrots, bouillon and harissa to a boil in a large pot and simmer until the vegetables are softened, about 20 minutes. Add the chick peas, cilantro and spinach and simmer until the spinach is wilted. Serve over brown rice or couscous. Each diner can stir in a little more harissa to suit his or her own taste.

4 to 6 servings

Spicy Eggplant Melange

Eggplant has a nice smokey taste if you char it first over an open gas flame or under a broiler.

>   2 eggplants
>   1 onion, chopped
>   2 cloves garlic, minced
>   1 cup bouillon (see page 187)
>   1 teaspoon Berbere spice mix (page 307) or to taste
>   3 ripe tomatoes, chopped
>   ½ cup curly vermicelli, crumbled
>   1 cup cooked brown rice
>   1 can chick peas, undrained, or 2 cups cooked
>   ½ cup golden raisins
>   ¼ cup lemon juice
>   ¼ cup Italian parsley, chopped
>   Freshly ground black pepper

Bring the onion, pepper, garlic, spices and bouillon to a boil in a medium saucepan. Simmer 5 to 10 minutes, or until the vegetables are softened. Add the beans, vinegar and pimentos and heat through.

4 to 6 servings

Black Beans with Tri-Color Vegetables

Rinsing the black beans doesn't change the taste of this dish, but it keeps the colors of the squash and carrots bright. Appearance counts!

> 1 onion, chopped
> 2 cloves garlic, minced
> 2 carrots, diced
> ½ cup bouillon (see page 187)
> 1 zucchini, diced
> 1 yellow squash, diced
> 2 cans black beans, drained and rinsed, or 3 cups cooked
> Juice of 2 limes
> 1 teaspoon cinnamon
> ½ teaspoon cumin
> ½ teaspoon turmeric
> 2 teaspoons curry powder
> Pinch cayenne or to taste
> Cooked brown rice

Bring the onion, garlic, carrots and bouillon to a boil in a medium saucepan. Simmer about 10 minutes, or until the carrots are just tender. Stir in the zucchini and yellow squash, black beans, lime juice and seasonings and cook 5 to 10 minutes, or until the squash is crisp-tender. Serve the bean mixture over the brown rice.

4 to 6 servings

Feijoida

This is my much-simplified and meat-free version of the national dish of Brazil. The real thing features several different cuts of meat, so calling this feijoida may be a bit of a stretch. I think the best parts of the feast are the black beans and rice, served with all the traditional garnishes.

Beans
1 onion, chopped
3 cloves garlic, minced
1 jalapeño pepper, chopped
1 can (28 ounces) plum tomatoes
3 cups cooked black beans or 2 cans, drained

Cook the onion, garlic and pepper in a little of the juice from the tomatoes 5 minutes. Add 1 cup of the beans and mash them well. Stir in the tomatoes, breaking them up. Add the rest of the beans and simmer 30 minutes.

Rice
1 cup brown rice
1 cup tomato juice
1½ cups bouillon (see page 187)

Bring the tomato juice and bouillon to a boil; stir in the rice, cover the pot and simmer 40 minutes, or until the rice is tender but not mushy.

Onions
2 onions, sliced thin
Boiling water to cover
3 tablespoons lime juice
1 teaspoon hot pepper sauce

Put the onions in a bowl, cover with boiling water and let stand 5 minutes; drain. Add the lime juice and the hot pepper sauce and marinate at least 30 minutes.

Greens
1 onion, chopped
½ cup water
1½ pounds chopped greens: kale, collards, spinach, Swiss chard, romaine lettuce, bok choy or any combination

In a large pot, bring the water to a boil; add the onion and simmer 5 minutes. Add the greens and cook until wilted but still tender (about 5 minutes for spinach, chard or lettuce, 15 to 20 for kale, collards or bok choy).

Oranges
4 oranges, peeled and sliced

Serve bowls of rice topped with the beans, and pass the greens, onions and oranges in separate bowls.

6 to 8 servings

Tamale Pie

The recipe for tamale pie must have appeared in a popular magazine in the 1950s, because I can remember when my mother started to make it and so can several of my friends. I'm sure it was touted as a way to "stretch a little hamburger to feed the whole family." No hamburger here, but the flavor brings back memories.

1 onion, chopped
4 cloves garlic, minced
1 green pepper, chopped
¼ cup bouillon (see page 187)
2 cans kidney beans, drained and mashed
¼ cup sliced black olives
2 tablespoons tomato paste
2 tablespoons chili powder
¼ cup Italian parsley, chopped

Crust
1 cup yellow cornmeal
1 tablespoon flour
2 teaspoons baking powder
¼ teaspoon salt
½ cup skim milk
1 can (4 ounces) chopped green chiles

Preheat the oven to 400°F. Bring the onion, garlic, green pepper and bouillon to a boil in a medium saucepan. Simmer 5 to 10 minutes or until the vegetables are soft. Stir in the beans, olives, tomato paste, chili powder and parsley and cook 5 minutes more. Spread the bean mixture in the bottom of an 8-inch baking dish. Combine the crust ingredients in a bowl, and spread over the bean mixture. Bake, uncovered, for 20 minutes.

6 to 8 servings

Tamale Stuffed Peppers

Stuffed peppers make a hearty meal for a cold winter day. You can steam them in a covered pot on your stovetop if you prefer.

> *4 large green peppers*
> *1 onion, chopped*
> *2 cloves garlic, minced*
> *½ cup bouillon (page 187)*
> *1 can (28 ounces) plum tomatoes, undrained*
> *1 tablespoon chili powder*
> *1 teaspoon ground cumin*
> *½ cup cornmeal*
> *1 can kidney beans, undrained*
> *1 cup fresh or frozen corn*
> *¼ cup sliced black olives*
> *Paprika*

Preheat the oven to 350° F. Cut the tops off the green peppers and remove the seeds and ribs. Blanch the peppers 5 minutes in a large pot of boiling water. Drain and set aside. Bring the onion, garlic and bouillon to a boil in a medium saucepan and simmer 5 minutes. Add the tomatoes, breaking them apart, and the spices. Stir in the cornmeal and cook 10 minutes, or until thick. Add the beans, corn and olives. Spoon the mixture into the peppers and sprinkle with paprika. Stand the peppers in a baking dish with ½ inch of water in the bottom. Bake 30 minutes.

4 servings

Easiest Baked Beans

These are best if you can cook them a day ahead to let the flavors blend. Refrigerate them and reheat before serving. If you can't wait, just dig in.

> 2 cans pinto beans, undrained
> 1 onion, chopped
> 1 cup ketchup
> ½ teaspoon salt
> ½ teaspoon ginger

Combine all ingredients in a medium saucepan, bring to a simmer and cook over very low heat 30 to 45 minutes, stirring occasionally.

4 servings

Cranberry Beans and Kale

If you think you don't like kale, try this recipe. It made a believer out of me.

> 1 onion, chopped
> 4 cloves garlic, minced
> 6 cups bouillon (see page 187)
> 1 pound cranberry beans or white beans, cooked, or 3 cans, undrained
> 1 can (6 ounces) tomato paste
> ½ teaspoon sage
> ½ teaspoon red pepper flakes
> 1 pound kale, chopped
> ½ cup cornmeal
> ½ cup water
> 2 tablespoons lemon juice
> Freshly ground black pepper

Bring the onion, garlic and ½ cup of the bouillon to a boil in a large pot and simmer until the vegetables are softened, about 10 minutes. Meanwhile, puree half of the beans in a blender. Add the remaining bouillon, pureed beans, whole beans, tomato paste, sage, red pepper flakes and kale to the pot; bring to a boil and simmer 30 minutes, or until the kale is tender. Mix the cornmeal, water and lemon juice into a paste and pour it slowly into the simmering stew, stirring constantly. Simmer 10 to 15 minutes. Serve with ground black pepper to taste.

6 to 8 servings

Pat's Bulgur and Lentils

Bulgur is wheat that has been steamed, then dried and crushed. Unlike other whole grains, it needs very little cooking time. You can prepare it for salads just by soaking it in water. In this spicy stew, you cook the bulgur and lentils together for a while to blend the flavors.

> 1 cup lentils
> 2 cups bouillon (see page 187)
> 1 onion, chopped
> 3 cloves garlic, minced
> 1 jalapeño pepper, seeded and minced
> 1 teaspoon ground cumin
> 1 cup bulgur
> ½ cup Italian parsley, chopped
> 2 tablespoons lemon juice
> Freshly ground black pepper

Cook the lentils in boiling water until just tender, about 20 minutes. Drain and set aside. Meanwhile, bring the bouillon to a boil and add the onion, garlic, pepper and cumin; simmer 10 minutes. Add the cooked lentils and bulgur, cover and simmer 20 to 25 minutes. Remove from the heat and let stand 10 minutes. Stir in the parsley and lemon juice and serve with ground black pepper to taste.

4 to 6 servings

Savoy Cabbage with Lentils

The wrinkly leaves of savoy cabbage give this lentil dish an interesting texture. You can make it with regular cabbage, too. Good over kasha or any whole grain.

> 1 cup orange lentils
> 5 cups bouillon, divided (see page 187)
> 1 onion, chopped
> 1 clove garlic, minced
> 1 head savoy cabbage, shredded
> 2 teaspoons mustard seed
> 1 teaspoon ground coriander
> 1 teaspoon turmeric
> Pinch cayenne or to taste

1 can (28 ounces) plum tomatoes, chopped
1 tablespoon lemon juice
Cooked kasha or other whole grain (optional)

Bring the lentils and 3 cups of the bouillon to a boil and simmer for 15 minutes. Meanwhile, in a second pot, bring the onion, garlic, cabbage and spices to a boil in the remaining 2 cups of bouillon and simmer 10 minutes. Add the tomatoes; return to boiling and simmer 30 minutes more. Stir in the lentils and the lemon juice and simmer 10 minutes. Serve over kasha if desired.

6 to 8 servings

Chick Pea Gumbo

Chick peas crop up everywhere in my recipes — in curries, soups, salads and pasta sauces. Here they are combined with okra and the other classic gumbo ingredients for a hearty dish with a southern flair.

1 onion, chopped
2 cloves garlic, minced
1 green pepper, chopped
1 can (28 ounces) plum tomatoes, chopped
1 dried red pepper, crumbled
¼ cup browned flour plus ¼ cup cold water (optional; see page 309)
1 pound okra, sliced
¼ cup parsley, chopped
¼ cup fresh basil leaves, chopped
1 bay leaf
2 cans chick peas, undrained
1 tablespoon lemon juice
Cooked brown rice

Bring the onion, garlic, pepper, tomatoes and their liquid, and the red pepper to a boil in a large pot and simmer 20 minutes. If you like a thick gumbo, stir the browned flour into the cold water and whisk it into the hot stew. Stir in the remaining ingredients and simmer 10 to15 minutes. Serve the gumbo over brown rice.

6 to 8 servings

Creole Sauce for Pasta or Rice

I can't claim that this is authentic Creole cooking, but it's one delicious sauce. If you're an okra fan, you'll love it. If you're not, this recipe just may convert you.

>1 onion, chopped
>1 green pepper, chopped
>1 can (28 ounces) plum tomatoes, chopped
>2 cups okra, sliced
>2 cups green beans, cut in 1-inch pieces
>½ cup Italian parsley, chopped
>¼ cup fresh basil leaves, chopped
>1 dried red pepper, crumbled
>1 can kidney beans, undrained
>Cooked pasta or brown rice

Cook the onion and green pepper in a little juice from the tomatoes 5 minutes. Add the tomatoes, okra, beans, parsley, basil and pepper and simmer 20 minutes. Stir in the kidney beans and serve over pasta or rice.

4 to 6 servings

Zesty Chick Pea Sauce

Quick and satisfying!

>2 cans chick peas, undrained
>1 can (28 ounces) plum tomatoes, chopped
>2 onions, sliced
>4 cloves garlic, minced
>1 teaspoon oregano
>1 dried red pepper, crumbled
>¼ cup Italian parsley, chopped
>Freshly ground black pepper
>Cooked whole grains or pasta

Puree one can of chick peas with their liquid in a blender. Bring the tomatoes to a boil in a large saucepan; add the onion, garlic, spices and pureed chick peas and simmer 15 minutes. Add the remaining can of chick peas and parsley. Serve over your favorite whole grain or pasta, with freshly ground pepper to taste.

4 to 6 servings

Marge's Lentil Pasta Sauce

This is a pasta sauce you can feed to the whole family. It's been known to fool children, teenagers and vegetable skeptics with its meaty texture.

> 1 onion, chopped
> 3 cloves garlic, minced
> 1 bay leaf
> 1 dried red pepper, crumbled
> 2 cups lentils
> 4 cups bouillon (see page 187)
> 2 cans (29 ounces each) tomato sauce
> 2 tablespoons fresh oregano or 2 teaspoons dried
> Cooked pasta or whole grains

Bring the onion, garlic, bay leaf, pepper, lentils and bouillon to a boil in a large pot. Simmer until the lentils are tender, 20 to 30 minutes. Drain off any excess liquid and stir in the tomato sauce and oregano; simmer 10 minutes. Serve over pasta or the grain of your choice.

6 to 8 servings

Asparagus Lasagna

My newsletter subscribers send me some very unusual and tasty recipes. I wondered about this one — until I tried it!

> 4½ cups bouillon, divided (see page 187)
> 1 cup brown rice
> 8 lasagna noodles
> 24 asparagus spears
> 2 cans chick peas, drained
> ¼ cup fresh basil leaves, chopped
> 1½ cups nonfat plain yogurt
> 5 tablespoons lemon juice
> 1 tablespoon cornstarch

Bring 2½ cups of the bouillon to a boil; add the brown rice and simmer until the rice is tender, about 40 minutes. Meanwhile, cook the lasagna noodles according to package directions; drain and set aside.

Break the tough ends off the asparagus and break the spears in half.

Steam them in ¼ inch of boiling water until crisp-tender, about 5 minutes (or use an electric steamer).

Puree the chick peas and basil in a blender with 1 cup of the yogurt; add 1 tablespoon of the lemon juice.

Stir the cornstarch into ¼ cup of cold bouillon. Heat the remaining bouillon and stir in the cornstarch mixture; simmer to thicken. Remove from the heat and stir in the remaining ½ cup of yogurt and 4 tablespoons of lemon juice.

Spoon a little of the bouillon mixture into the bottom of a 9-by-13-inch glass baking dish, then cover it with 4 of the lasagna noodles. Spread the pureed chick peas on the noodles. Place the asparagus on the chick pea mixture, then spread the cooked rice over the asparagus. Top with the 4 remaining noodles. Gently pour the remaining broth mixture over the noodles. Heat, uncovered, in a microwave oven 5 minutes, or until piping hot.

4 to 6 servings

Stan's Pasta e Fagioli

Stan loves Italian food. This is his version of the Old Country favorite, and he says it tastes as good as the high-fat original.

> 1 onion, chopped
> 2 carrots, sliced
> 2 celery stalks, sliced
> 3 cloves garlic, minced
> 1 can (28 ounces) plum tomatoes, chopped
> ¼ teaspoon red pepper flakes
> 1 pound spinach, chopped
> 2 small zucchini, sliced
> 1 can cannellini or white beans, undrained, or 2 cups cooked
> ¼ cup Italian parsley, chopped
> ¼ cup fresh basil leaves, chopped
> 1 tablespoon fresh oregano leaves, chopped, or 1 teaspoon dried
> 1 pound pasta shells or other small shape
> Freshly ground black pepper

Bring the onion, carrot, celery, garlic, tomatoes and the red pepper flakes to a boil in a large pot. Simmer until the vegetables are softened, about 10 minutes. Add the spinach, zucchini, beans, parsley, basil and oregano and cook 15 to 20 minutes. Meanwhile, cook the pasta until *al dente* (tender but chewy) and drain. Mix the cooked pasta into the vegetables and serve with ground pepper to taste.

4 to 6 servings

Quick Southwestern Beans and Pasta

Here's another favorite recipe from a *Mirkin Report* subscriber. My readers have good taste!

> 1 onion, sliced
> 1 sweet red pepper, chopped
> ¼ cup bouillon (see page 187)
> 1 can pinto beans, drained
> 1 can (4 ounces) chopped green chiles, drained
> 1 cup frozen corn
> 2 teaspoons chili powder
> 2 tablespoons cilantro leaves, chopped
> 3 cups cooked shells or other small pasta

Bring the onion, pepper and bouillon to a boil in a medium saucepan; simmer about 5 minutes, or until the vegetables are softened. Stir in the remaining ingredients and heat through.

4 to 6 servings

Fiery Lentil-Rice-Macaroni Combo

This is as bland as they come until you stir in the harissa. I like mine hot! Add a little at a time and taste as you go.

> 1 cup brown rice
> 5½ cups bouillon, divided (see page 187)
> 2 cups lentils
> 1 onion, chopped
> ½ cup macaroni
> 1 teaspoon harissa (page 307) or to taste

Bring the rice and 2½ cups of bouillon to a boil and simmer, covered, 45 minutes, or until rice is tender but not mushy. Meanwhile, cook the lentils and onion in the remaining 3 cups of bouillon until tender, 20 to 30 minutes. At the same time, cook the macaroni according to the package directions until *al dente*; rinse in cold water and drain. Combine the brown rice, lentils and macaroni and stir in the harissa.

6 to 8 servings

Bajan Beans and Rice

This may be my prettiest bean and rice recipe, with bright bits of red and green pepper, corn and cilantro leaves in a rosy brew. True fans of the food of Barbados will want to add several dashes of hot pepper sauce.

> 1 onion, chopped
> 2 cloves garlic, minced
> 1 green pepper, chopped
> 1 sweet red pepper, chopped
> 1 jalapeño pepper, sliced
> 3 cups bouillon (see page 187)
> 3 fresh or canned tomatoes, chopped
> 1 acorn squash, peeled and cubed
> 1 cup brown rice
> 3 cups cooked small white beans or 2 cans, undrained
> 1 cup frozen corn
> ¼ cup cilantro, chopped
> 1 tablespoon capers
> Hot pepper sauce to taste

Bring the onion, garlic, green, red and jalapeño peppers and ½ cup of the bouillon to a boil in a large pot. Simmer 10 minutes, or until the vegetables are softened. Add the remaining bouillon, tomatoes, squash and rice. Return to a boil; reduce the heat and simmer, covered, 45 minutes, or until the rice is tender. Stir in the beans, corn, cilantro, capers and hot sauce and heat through, about 5 minutes. Serve with the hot pepper sauce on the table so each person can adjust the heat to his or her liking.

6 to 8 servings

Main Dishes with Seafood

I recommend that you eat fish or shellfish 3 to 4 times a week. Of course, you do not add any fat while cooking it, so that means no fried fish and no basting with butter while you broil it. The recipes in this section will show you dozens of delicious ways to prepare seafood main dishes without any added fat.

Seafood is an excellent source of protein, minerals and other nutrients. However, it is low in fiber, so you should limit the amount you eat at a meal. The number of servings indicated with each of these recipes is based on a quarter pound of seafood per portion.

Always buy seafood to take advantage of the freshest, best-looking varieties in your fish market. You can substitute different kinds of fish and shellfish in most of these recipes.

Happy fishing!

Shrimp Jambalaya

Shrimp is a quick-cooking, low-fat treat, and I'm always trying new ways to serve it. This zesty jambalaya is one of my favorites.

> 1 pound shrimp
> 3 cups bouillon (see page 187)
> 1 bay leaf
> 1 onion, chopped
> 1 green pepper, chopped
> 3 stalks celery, chopped
> 2 cloves garlic, minced
> 1 can (28 ounces) plum tomatoes, chopped
> 1 cup brown rice
> 1 tablespoon hot pepper sauce
> ½ teaspoon thyme
> 6 green onions, chopped
> ¼ cup Italian parsley, chopped
> Freshly ground black pepper

Peel the shrimp and set aside. Bring the shrimp shells, bouillon and bay leaf to a boil and simmer 20 minutes while chopping the vegetables. Strain the bouillon and return to the pot. Add the onion, pepper, celery, garlic, tomatoes, rice, hot sauce and thyme to the bouillon and simmer 45 minutes, or until the rice is tender. Stir in the shrimp, green onion and parsley and cook 2 to 3 minutes, or until the shrimp are pink and firm. Serve with ground pepper to taste.

4 servings

Seafood Paella

My low-fat paella is a gourmet treat — great party fare served with a green salad and crusty French bread. You can vary the shellfish and fish based on what looks good at your market. Try ½ pound of squid cut in rings in place of ½ pound of the fish.

> 1 onion, chopped
> 1 green pepper, chopped
> 2½ cups bouillon (see page 187)
> 1 cup brown rice
> 1 can (28 ounces) plum tomatoes, chopped
> 1 teaspoon red pepper flakes or to taste
> ½ teaspoon ground coriander
> ½ teaspoon saffron
> 1 teaspoon oregano
> 1 bay leaf
> 1 pound flounder or other firm white fish fillet, cut in 2-inch pieces
> 16 mussels or cherrystone clams
> ½ pound shrimp, peeled
> 1 cup frozen green peas, thawed
> Italian parsley, chopped

Bring the onion, pepper and bouillon to a boil in a large pot and simmer 5 minutes. Add the rice, tomatoes and seasonings and simmer, covered, about 40 minutes, or until the rice is tender. Stir the fish pieces into the rice. Place the mussels or clams on top of the rice; cover and steam just until the shells open. Discard any that fail to open. Stir in the shrimp and cook just until the shrimp turn pink — about 3 minutes. Stir in the peas and sprinkle with parsley.

6 servings

Cajun Fish Fillets

The flavor comes close to those wonderful "blackened" fish dishes without all the fat.

> 1 pound orange roughy or any firm white fish fillets
> 1 teaspoon Cajun spice (such as McCormick or Paul Prudhomme)
> 1 tablespoon paprika
> Lemon wedges
> Freshly ground black pepper

Preheat the broiler. Arrange the fillets on a broiler pan lined with aluminum foil. Combine the Cajun spice and paprika and dust heavily on the fillets. Broil close to the flame 5 to 6 minutes, or until the spices are browned and the fish is firm and flakes with a fork. Serve with lemon wedges and ground pepper to taste.

4 servings

Poached Fish with Ginger

This is a basic fish cooking technique that works with many other combinations of bottom-layer vegetables, seasonings and garnishes. You can serve the "steaming rack" vegetables, or use tough outer leaves or stalks and discard them.

> 3 or 4 stalks of celery, cut into sticks
> 1-inch piece of gingerroot, minced
> 1 clove garlic, minced
> 1 lemon, sliced
> ¼ cup soy sauce
> 1 cup water
> 1 pound flounder or other lean white fish fillets
> Italian parsley, chopped

Arrange the celery sticks in a layer in the bottom of a covered saucepan. This is your "steaming rack." Add the next 5 ingredients; bring to a boil and simmer 5 minutes. Lay the fish on the celery; cover the pan and steam about 5 minutes, or until the fish flakes with a fork. Sprinkle with chopped parsley.

4 servings

Baked Fillets with Mushrooms, Shallots and Dill

Using this simple method, fish stays moist and flavorful. With portobello or other "fancy" mushrooms, it's gourmet fare for guests, but it's almost as delicious with ordinary mushrooms and a little chopped mild onion or green onions. You can substitute virtually any fresh tender herb for the dill — oregano, marjoram or even parsley. The recipe can be easily doubled or tripled to serve a crowd.

> 1 pound firm white fish fillets (such as orange roughy)
> 1/4 pound portobello mushrooms (or other variety of your choice), sliced
> 1/4 pound shallots, peeled and chopped
> 1/4 cup fresh dill, snipped
> Juice of 1 lemon
> Freshly ground black pepper

Preheat the oven to 450° F. Spread half of the mushrooms and half of the shallots in the bottom of an 8-by-13-inch glass pan or nonstick metal baking pan. Lay the fillets over the vegetables in a single layer. Sprinkle the remaining mushrooms and shallots and the snipped dill over the fillets. Squeeze the lemon juice over the fish and grind on fresh black pepper to taste. Cover the dish with foil and seal the edges tightly. Bake 15 to 20 minutes, or until the fish flakes easily with a fork.

Alternative cooking method: This recipe works beautifully in a clay cooker. Follow the directions that come with your cooker for presoaking; arrange the ingredients inside and place the cooker in a cold oven. Turn the heat up to 450°F. and cook 30 minutes.

4 servings

Crab Delight

Bright red and green vegetables make this delightful to look at as well as to taste. You could easily substitute shrimp or scallops for the crab meat.

> 1 sweet red pepper, chopped
> 4 green onions, minced
> 2 tablespoons grated fresh gingerroot
> Juice of 1 lemon

2 ripe tomatoes
¼ pound mushrooms, chopped
1 can water chestnuts, diced
1 cup broccoli florets
¼ pound snow peas
1 pound crab meat or surimi (see page 172)
Freshly ground black pepper
Cooked brown rice or toasted pita breads (optional)

In a medium saucepan, cook the pepper, onion and gingerroot in the lemon juice to soften, about 5 minutes. Cut the tomatoes in half and squeeze the pulp and juice into the pan. Add the mushrooms, water chestnuts and broccoli; cover and steam about 10 minutes, or until the broccoli is crisp-tender. Add the snow peas and crab meat and cook 2 to 3 minutes. Serve over brown rice or as a pita bread sandwich filling, with ground pepper to taste.

4 servings

Baked Flounder and Vegetables

Baking fish fillets in a foil-covered dish is a foolproof technique that is fancy enough to serve to company. Once you have tried this recipe, you can work out endless variations: use any firm white fish and any combination of vegetables you like. You can use different spices and even different cooking liquids — bouillon, clam juice or tomato juice work well.

2 small zucchini, cut into matchsticks
2 carrots, cut into matchsticks
2 onions, sliced
Juice of 4 lemons
1 tablespoon curry powder
1 cup plum tomatoes, chopped
1 pound flounder fillets
1¼ cups dry white wine (optional)
1 cup Italian parsley, chopped
Freshly ground black pepper

Preheat the oven to 450°F. Blanch the zucchini and carrot strips in boiling water for 1 minute; drain and set aside. Cook the onions in a little of the lemon juice until softened, about 5 minutes; add the remaining juice, curry powder, tomatoes and wine and cook over high heat 5 to 7

About Surimi

Have you discovered surimi? Surimi is made from low-fat fish, usually pollack, that is flavored to taste like crab or lobster. You may not believe you're eating the real thing, but it is very inexpensive and quite tasty.

The flavor of these imitation crab and lobster products varies widely. Some of them are excellent, while others are boring at best. I've also noticed that the prices range widely as well, and the more expensive ones don't necessarily taste better. Try different brands that are offered in your supermarket until you find one or two that you like. Keep your eye out for specials; sometimes my store practically gives surimi away.

I've included several recipes that use surimi or list surimi as an optional ingredient. You can substitute surimi in any seafood salad. In soups or other hot seafood dishes, be sure to add the surimi at the very end; it should only be warmed through or cooked for a few minutes at the most. Because it is made from fish that has been pulverized into a paste, surimi breaks down quickly if it is cooked too long.

minutes; remove from the heat, and stir in the carrots, zucchini and parsley. Arrange the fillets in a baking dish; spoon the vegetable mixture over the fish and seal the dish with aluminum foil. Bake 15 minutes, or until the fish flakes with a fork. Serve with ground black pepper to taste.

4 servings

North Country Scallops

The best time to cook with apples is in the fall, when they are nice and crisp and tart. You can pare them if you like; I never do.

> 1/2 cup fish stock (see page 187)
> 1/4 cup dry white wine (optional)
> 2 teaspoons grated fresh gingerroot
> 1/2 teaspoon freshly ground black pepper
> 2 apples, cored and diced
> 1 pound scallops
> 2 cups cooked wild rice

Bring the stock, wine, gingerroot and pepper to a boil in a medium saucepan; stir in the apples and cook 5 minutes, or until the apples are barely soft. Add the scallops and simmer 2 minutes. Serve over wild rice with additional ground black pepper to taste.

4 servings

Fish Fillets with Ginger Marmalade Sauce

If you can find ginger marmalade — a British favorite — try it in this recipe. You won't need any additional ginger.

> ½ cup orange marmalade
> 1 tablespoon grated gingerroot or 1 teaspoon dried ginger
> 3 tablespoons Dijon mustard
> 1 tablespoon vinegar
> 1 pound turbot or any firm white fish fillets

Combine the marmalade, gingerroot, mustard and vinegar. Spread a little of the sauce on each fillet and broil 5 to 6 minutes, or until the fish flakes with a fork. Serve with the remaining sauce.

4 servings

Pasta with Mussels

Farm-raised mussels are available year-round. This recipe is easy enough for a quick supper and fancy enough for a party.

> 4 pounds mussels
> 1 cup clam juice or white wine
> 4 cloves garlic, minced
> 1 onion, minced
> 1 can (28 ounces) plum tomatoes, chopped
> 1 tablespoon fresh oregano or 1 teaspoon dried
> ½ teaspoon red pepper flakes
> Cooked pasta

Sort through the mussels and discard any that stay open when you handle them or that have badly broken shells. Scrub them and remove their beards. Bring the juice or wine to a boil in a large pot; add the mussels, cover and steam until the shells open. Discard any that fail to open. Cool and remove the meat from the shells. Strain the cooking liquid if it's gritty, and set aside.

Bring the garlic, onion, tomatoes, oregano and pepper flakes to a boil and simmer 20 to 30 minutes. Add the mussels and their cooking liquid; simmer 5 minutes and serve over cooked fettuccine or other pasta.

4 servings

Mussels with Tomatoes and Basil

This is an even simpler way to serve mussels, perfect for summertime when you can get vine-ripened tomatoes and fresh basil — perhaps from your own garden. Serve with warm French bread to soak up the delicious sauce.

> 4 pounds mussels
> 1 cup dry white wine
> 2 cloves garlic, minced
> 6 ripe tomatoes, peeled and chopped (or use canned plum tomatoes)
> 1 cup fresh basil leaves, chopped
> Freshly ground black pepper

Scrub the mussels and remove their beards. Discard any with cracked or open shells. Bring the wine, garlic and tomatoes to a boil in a large pot; add the mussels and steam, covered, until their shells open. Stir in the basil and ground pepper to taste.

4 servings

Stan's Fettuccine Marinara

This fettuccine is so delicious you'll want a big serving. Count one bowlful as two portions of seafood — and enjoy!

> 2 onions, chopped
> 1 green pepper, chopped
> 6 green onions, chopped
> 4 cloves garlic, minced
> 1 cup dry white wine
> 2 cans (28 ounces each) plum tomatoes, chopped
> 3 cups clam juice
> 2 bay leaves

¼ teaspoon red pepper flakes
1 tablespoon fresh oregano or 1 teaspoon dried
18 mussels, cleaned
18 small clams, cleaned
1 pound shrimp, peeled
1 pound scallops
1 cup fresh basil leaves, chopped
Cooked fettuccine

Bring the onion, pepper, green onions, garlic and wine to a boil in a large pot. Simmer about 10 minutes, or until the vegetables are softened. Add the tomatoes, clam juice, bay leaves, red pepper flakes and oregano and simmer 15 to 20 minutes. Add the mussels and clams and cook until the shells begin to open. Discard any that do not open. Stir in the shrimp and scallops and cook 2 to 3 minutes, or just until the shrimp are pink and firm. Add the basil leaves and serve over cooked fettuccine.

6 to 8 servings
Each serving counts as 2 portions of seafood.

Seafarer's Stew

This hearty stew can be made with any combination of fish or shellfish; just pick out the best that's available in your fish market. As with Stan's Fettuccine Marinara, you'll probably eat more than 4 ounces of seafood in one sitting.

2 onions, chopped
4 cloves garlic, minced
4 stalks celery, sliced
1 cup clam juice
2 cans (28 ounces each) plum tomatoes, chopped
2 carrots, chopped
2 potatoes, diced
Pinch cayenne or to taste
1 pound shrimp, peeled
1 pound scallops
1 pound haddock or any firm white fish fillets
1 can (6½ ounces) chopped clams
12 ounces crab meat or surimi
½ cup white wine or sherry
Juice of 1 lemon
Freshly ground black pepper

Bring the onion, garlic, celery and clam juice to a boil in a large pot. Simmer about 10 minutes, or until the vegetables are softened. Add the tomatoes, carrots, potatoes and cayenne and simmer 20 minutes. Stir in the seafood, wine and lemon juice, and continue to simmer for 10 to 15 minutes. Serve with ground black pepper to taste.

6 to 8 servings
Each serving counts as 2 portions of seafood.

Italian Sole

Seasoned tomatoes broil along with the fish, and their juice keeps the fish nice and moist.

> 1 pound sole or other firm white fish fillets
> Paprika
> 2 cloves garlic, minced
> 3 ripe fresh tomatoes, chopped
> 1/4 cup fresh basil leaves, chopped
> Lemon wedges
> Freshly ground black pepper

Preheat the broiler. Place the fillets on a foil-covered broiler pan and sprinkle with paprika. Mix the garlic, tomatoes and basil together and spread over the fish. Broil 5 to 6 minutes, or until the fish is firm and the tomatoes are slightly browned. Garnish with lemon wedges and grind on pepper to taste.

4 servings

Clam and Mushroom Sauce for Grains or Pasta

For variety, you can serve this garlicy clam sauce over spaghetti squash (see page 198).

> 1 onion, chopped
> 2 cloves garlic, minced
> 1/2 cup bouillon (see page 187)
> 1 can (29 ounces) tomato sauce

1 tablespoon fresh oregano or ½ teaspoon dried
1 bay leaf
¼ teaspoon red pepper flakes
½ pound mushrooms, sliced
2 cans (6½ ounces) chopped clams
Freshly ground black pepper
Cooked pasta or whole grains

Bring the onion, garlic and bouillon to a boil in a medium saucepan, and simmer 5 minutes. Add the tomato sauce and seasonings and simmer 10 minutes. Add the mushrooms and clams with their juice, and simmer 10 minutes. Serve over whole grains, pasta or spaghetti squash, with ground black pepper to taste.

Enough sauce for 4 to 6 bowls of pasta or grains

Squid Sauce for Grains or Pasta

If you've never tried squid, please be brave and do it now. It's fun! Squid is chewy and quite bland, absorbing all the flavor of the sauce you cook it in. The rings curl attractively as soon as they hit the hot liquid, and the tentacles look like creatures from a science fiction movie. Kids love them. Sometimes you can buy cleaned squid at the fish counter, but it's easy and much more economical to clean it yourself.

1 3-pound box of frozen squid or 1½ pounds cleaned
2 onions, chopped
3 cloves garlic, minced
1 cup bottled clam juice
1 can (28 ounces) tomato sauce
1 teaspoon oregano
¼ teaspoon thyme
½ teaspoon red pepper flakes
Freshly ground black pepper
Cooked whole grains or pasta

If you are using frozen squid, thaw, clean and cut it according to the directions on page 178. If you purchase cleaned squid from your fish market, slice the body sacs crossways into ¼-inch rings. Set aside.

Cook the onion and garlic in a little of the clam juice to soften, 5 to 10 minutes. Add the remaining juice, tomato sauce and seasonings and simmer 15 minutes. Stir in the squid and cook 3 to 5 minutes, until the squid rings curl. Do not overcook or the squid will toughen. Serve over your favorite whole grain or pasta, with ground black pepper to taste.

6 to 8 servings

Fettuccine with Shrimp Sauce

Large butterflied shrimp are impressive, but any size will work fine. Small ones are quicker to prepare — just peel them and use them uncut.

> *2 pounds large shrimp*
> *1 onion, chopped*

Cleaning Squid

Squid comes frozen in 3-pound blocks. Thaw it in your refrigerator or in cold water. To clean squid, you will need a cutting board, a sharp knife and a bowl. A 3-pound box yields about 1½ pounds of cleaned squid body sacs and tentacles.

- Pull the tentacles gently from the body sac. The squid innards should come out of the body. Set the body sac aside.
- Cut the tentacles off just above the eyes. Don't be surprised if you puncture the ink sac, squirting a little dark purple liquid.
- Remove the beak-like piece from the center of the tentacles and discard. Put the tentacles in the bowl, and discard the rest of the head and innards.
- Remove the stiff, transparent "quill" from inside the body sac and discard. If you can feel more innards inside the body sac, squeeze it from the bottom up, push out and discard any jelly-like matter.
- Peel the speckled skin off the body sac and discard.
- Pull the triangular "fins" off the sides of the body sac and place them in the bowl.
- Slice the body sac into ¼- to ½-inch rings and place them in the bowl. If you are preparing very large squid, you may want to cut the tentacles and the triangular flaps into pieces, but they are usually small enough to cook whole.
- Proceed to the next squid. After you get the hang of it, you may want to work assembly-line style: remove the innards and cut off the tentacles of all the squid; then clean all the body sacs; then do all the slicing.

---

3 cloves garlic, minced
¼ cup Italian parsley, chopped
¼ teaspoon red pepper flakes
1 tablespoon fresh oregano or 1 teaspoon dried
½ cup clam juice or bouillon (see page 187)
½ cup dry white wine
Cooked fettuccine
Freshly ground black pepper

Preheat the broiler. Peel and butterfly the shrimp (split them down the middle, not all the way through, and open up like the pages of a book). Place the shrimp in a single layer in a foil-lined broiling pan.

Cook the onion, garlic, parsley, red pepper flakes and oregano in the

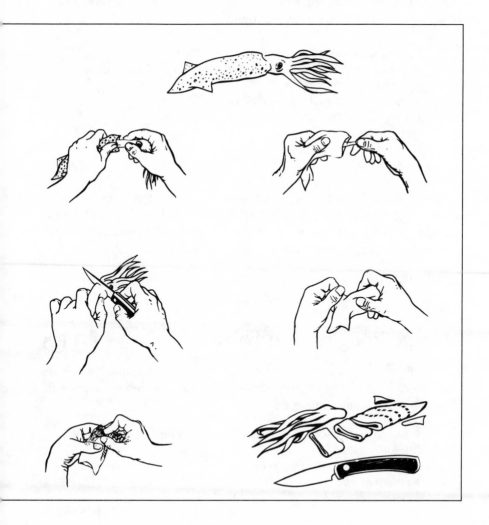

clam juice or bouillon until soft, about 5 minutes. Stir in the wine and pour the mixture over the shrimp. Broil for 3 minutes about 4 inches from the heat, or until the shrimp are pink and firm. Divide the fettuccine into serving dishes and spoon the shrimp and some of the juice over each portion. Serve with ground black pepper to taste.

6 to 8 servings

Seafood Kabobs

Kabobs can be cooked on an outdoor grill or under a broiler. You might want to make some all-vegetable or fruit kabobs at the same time. Don't overcook the shrimp; they dry out quickly.

> *1 pound medium shrimp, peeled*
> *1 pound halibut steaks or other firm white fish, cut in 1-inch cubes*
> *½ pound sea scallops*
> *2 cups fresh or canned pineapple chunks*
> *1 pound cherry tomatoes*
> *Lemon wedges*
> *Freshly ground black pepper*
> *Cooked wild rice (optional)*

Arrange the seafood, pineapple chunks and cherry tomatoes on wood skewers. Squeeze lemon juice over each kabob and broil or grill 5 to 8 minutes, turning 3 or 4 times. Serve with additional lemon wedges and ground black pepper to taste, over wild rice if desired.

6 to 8 servings

Orange Roughy with Salsa

Orange roughy is one of my favorite low-fat fishes for broiling because its own juices keep it from drying out — as long as you don't overcook it. This is a nice summertime dish.

> *1 pound orange roughy or other firm white fish fillets*
> *Paprika*
> *Freshly ground black pepper to taste*
> *1 tablespoon vinegar*
> *2 cloves garlic, minced*

2 large, ripe tomatoes, chopped
6 green onions, sliced
1 tablespoon lemon juice
1 jalapeño pepper, minced

Sprinkle the fillets with paprika and pepper to taste and broil 5 minutes, or until the fish is opaque and flakes easily with a fork. Arrange the fish on a serving platter and sprinkle with vinegar. Chill for 20 minutes. Meanwhile, mix the remaining ingredients to make the salsa. Pour the salsa over the fillets and serve at room temperature.

4 servings

Baked Whole Flounder with Swiss Chard

This recipe for baked whole fish can be varied endlessly. Any low-fat fish and just about any vegetables and seasonings can be used. You can also steam the fish on the stovetop, if desired.

2 large bunches Swiss chard, cut in 3-inch pieces
4 cloves garlic, minced
1 large onion, chopped
1 can (28 ounces) plum tomatoes, chopped
1 whole flounder or any firm white fish, 3 to 4 pounds
Freshly ground pepper to taste

Preheat the oven to 400° F. Pour half the tomatoes into a covered pan or casserole large enough to hold the fish. (Or use an open pan with a foil cover.) Spread half of the Swiss chard, garlic and onions on the tomatoes. Add the fish and sprinkle with pepper. Cover with the remaining tomatoes, garlic and onions. Bake, covered, 20 minutes. Remove the cover, spoon some of the sauce over the fish and bake another 5 to 10 minutes.

4 to 6 servings

Oyster and Shrimp Gumbo

Most of the time I'm content with my vegetarian gumbos. Once in a while, I indulge myself with this deluxe version with oysters and shrimp. This is a perfect dish for any of the holidays that fall in oyster season — months with an *r* in them.

1 pint shucked oysters and their liquid
1 pound medium shrimp
4 cups fish stock or bouillon (see page 187)
2 bay leaves
1 onion, chopped
5 cloves garlic, minced
1 green pepper, chopped
2 stalks celery, chopped
¼ cup browned flour (see page 309)
1 can (28 ounces) plum tomatoes, chopped
½ cup Italian parsley, chopped
1 teaspoon hot pepper sauce or to taste
2 teaspoons fresh thyme or ½ teaspoon dried
1 teaspoon fennel seeds
3 cups okra, cut in ½-inch pieces
Freshly ground black pepper
Cooked brown rice

Drain the oysters and set them aside; add their liquid to the stock. Peel the shrimp and set aside; add their shells to the stock. Bring the stock to a boil with the bay leaves and cook 15 minutes. Strain the stock; return ½ cup to the pot and reserve the rest.

Bring the onion, garlic, green pepper, celery and ½ cup of the stock to a boil in a large pot and simmer 10 minutes, or until the vegetables are softened.

Meanwhile, place another ½ cup of the stock in a small bowl; stir in 2 or 3 ice cubes to chill. Remove any unmelted ice and stir in the browned flour to form a thick paste.

Add the flour mixture, tomatoes, parsley, hot pepper sauce, thyme and fennel to the pot and simmer for 20 minutes, stirring occasionally. Add the okra and simmer 5 minutes. Add shrimp and oysters and cook just until the shrimp are pink and the oyster edges are curled, about 5 minutes. Serve over brown rice, with ground pepper and additional hot pepper sauce to taste.

8 servings

Brown Rice Sushi

I don't recommend eating raw fish because of possible parasites, but there are many possibilities for low-fat sushi using cooked seafood. Brown rice doesn't stick together as well as the traditional short-grain white rice, but it gives you more fiber. Your creations may not look like those of a professional sushi chef (they practice for years), but the wonderful flavors are there. Follow these basic directions, and then try your own variations.

> *Cooked brown rice*
> *Rice wine vinegar**
> *Ssteamed shrimp, crab meat or sea crab sticks*
> *Cucumber*
> *Nori sheets (dried seaweed)**
> *Wasabi**
> *Soy sauce*
> *Pickled ginger**
>
> ** Available in Asian grocery stores and in the Asian section of many supermarkets.*

Moisten a cup of cooked brown rice with about 2 tablespoons of rice wine vinegar.

Mix about 3 tablespoons of wasabi powder with enough water to make a paste. Slice the cucumber into matchstick-size pieces.

Briefly toast a sheet of nori over a gas flame. Set it on a bamboo sushi rolling mat or a piece of wax paper. Pat on a thin layer of rice (about ¼ inch), leaving about ½ inch of the seaweed showing on each side.

Smear a small amount of wasabi in a thin strip down the middle of the rice. (Start with just a little — it's horseradish-hot.)

Arrange a strip of crab meat or shrimp pieces and some of the cucumber sticks down the center. Roll up tightly and moisten the edge of the nori to seal. Slice in 1-inch pieces. Repeat with remaining ingredients.

Accompany each serving with small dishes of soy sauce for dipping and little mounds of wasabi and pickled ginger. Each person can add wasabi to the soy sauce to taste.

1 serving equals 4 ounces of seafood

Fillets in Green Chile Salsa

I'm often asked how to keep broiled fish from drying out when you can't baste it with butter. In this recipe, the marinated fillets stay nice and moist, and the flavor is extraordinary. Check the fish often as it broils to make sure you don't overcook it.

> 1 pound halibut or other firm white fish fillets
> 5 mild green chiles, roasted, peeled, seeded and chopped, or 2 cans
>   (4 ounces each) chopped green chiles (see page 138)
> 2 cloves garlic, minced
> ¼ cup lemon juice
> ¼ cup cilantro, chopped
> ½ teaspoon ground coriander
> Paprika
> ½ cup fish stock (see page 187)
> Freshly ground black pepper
> Lemon wedges

Place the fish in a glass or plastic dish (not metal). Mix the chiles, garlic, lemon juice, cilantro and coriander and pour over the fish. Marinate several hours or overnight. Remove the fish from the marinade; place it on a foil-covered broiling pan, sprinkle with paprika and broil 5 to 6 minutes, or until it flakes with a fork. Mix the marinade and stock in a small pot; bring it to a boil and simmer 5 minutes. Pour the sauce over the fish, add ground black pepper to taste and serve with lemon wedges.

4 servings

Flying Fish

You may not have freshly caught flying fish, but with a little imagination you can conjure up salty Caribbean breezes to go with this feast.

> 1 onion, chopped
> 1 green pepper, chopped
> 1 or 2 fresh hot chiles (such as jalapeños), chopped
> 2 cloves garlic, minced
> 1 cup chopped, peeled tomatoes, fresh or canned

2 tablespoons cilantro leaves, chopped
1/4 cup lime juice
1 cup fish stock or clam juice (see page 187)
2 pounds haddock or other firm white fish fillets, cut in large chunks
Cooked brown rice (optional)
Black beans (optional — see page 141)
Hot pepper sauce

Puree the onion, peppers, garlic, tomatoes, cilantro, lime juice and about 1/4 cup of the stock in a blender until smooth. Heat the sauce to boiling in a small pan and simmer 10 minutes, stirring frequently. Allow the sauce to cool and pour it over the fillets in a large pot. Refrigerate the fish for at least 1 hour. Stir the remaining stock into the pot, heat to boiling and simmer gently until the fish flakes, 6 to 10 minutes. Serve over brown rice with a side dish of black beans. Pass the hot sauce so each diner can add his or her own "island heat."

8 servings

West African Seafood Stew

I think every country with an ocean coastline has developed its own version of a seafood stew, and I love them all. The sweet potatoes and green bananas make this one special. It's supposed to be very spicy, but you may want to add a little of the cayenne at a time and taste as you go.

3 cups fish stock (see page 187)
1 pound shrimp, unshelled
4 onions, chopped
4 garlic cloves, minced
1/2 teaspoon cayenne or to taste
1/4 teaspoon thyme
2 potatoes, diced
2 sweet potatoes, peeled and diced
2 cups cabbage, chopped
1 can (28 ounces) plum tomatoes, chopped
1 cup Italian parsley, chopped
1 pound flounder fillets or any firm white fish
2 green unripe bananas, sliced
Lemon or lime wedges

Bring the stock to a boil in a large pot and drop in the shrimp; cook for 2 minutes, remove with a slotted spoon and set aside to cool. Add the onion, garlic, spices, potatoes, sweet potatoes, cabbage, tomatoes and parsley to the stock and simmer for 15 minutes, or until the potatoes are just tender. Meanwhile, peel the shrimp and cut the fish into 2-inch chunks. Add fish and banana slices to the stew and cook 10 minutes more. Stir in the shrimp and serve with lemon or lime wedges.

8 servings

Hearty Soups with Vegetables, Grains and Beans

These soups are main dishes that you serve in bowls. With a salad and perhaps some bread, you have a whole meal. Whole grains, beans and starchy vegetables are natural thickeners, so you can create hearty, satisfying soups without a trace of added fat.

All of the soups in this section freeze well. It's so easy to make a large quantity that you may want to double your favorite recipes. Soups often taste even better the second day, after the flavors have had time to blend.

These hearty soups are ideal for lunch, too. Take a thermos to work or heat up a container in the office microwave. For lunch or dinner, soups are a mainstay of your low-fat diet. You'll never run out of great-tasting combinations of vegetables, grains, beans and spices.

Great Veggie Soup

The beauty of this recipe — as with most vegetable soups — is the freedom to add and subtract ingredients based on what looks good in the produce department. Add long-cooking vegetables in the beginning, short-cooking vegetables at the end. Make lots — soup often tastes better the next day, and it freezes well.

> 1 large onion, chopped
> 4 carrots, sliced
> 4 cloves garlic, minced
> 1/2 cup lentils
> 8 cups bouillon (see page 187)
> 1 bay leaf

¼ teaspoon cayenne pepper or to taste
1 teaspoon ground coriander
2 cups red potatoes, unpeeled and cut in ½-inch dice
1 can (28 ounces) Italian plum tomatoes, chopped
1 can chick peas, undrained
2 cans artichoke hearts, drained and quartered
¼ cup Italian parsley, chopped
1 lemon, cut in wedges
Freshly ground black pepper

Bring the first eight ingredients to a boil in a large pot, and simmer for 10 minutes. Add the potatoes and cook 20 minutes longer, or until the potatoes are tender. Add the tomatoes, chick peas, artichoke hearts and parsley, and simmer 5 minutes. Ladle into bowls and serve with lemon wedges and freshly ground pepper to taste.

6 to 8 servings

About Bouillon and Stock

You'll notice that lots of my recipes list **bouillon** as an ingredient. That's my shorthand for using a flavored liquid instead of water. Chapter 8 explains why flavored liquids are so important in low-fat recipes. When one of my recipes calls for bouillon, here's what to use:

Bouillon cubes or granules. The easiest method is to add *one bouillon cube or one teaspoon of bouillon granules for each 1 to 2 cups of water.* I use chicken bouillon cubes all the time because they are so convenient. Use vegetable flavor if you prefer, or beef flavor in hearty recipes such as chilies.

Dashi or powdered fish stock. These are similar to bouillon granules but with a fish flavor. Asian grocery stores are your best source — they have dozens of varieties, usually in foil packets or little jars. Use these wherever a recipe calls for fish stock or where you want a fish flavor.

Homemade stock. Classic chefs swear by homemade stock, and believe that canned bouillon or bouillon cubes are mortal sins. I'm not such a purist. Sometimes I make my own, but I must admit that I usually don't. The traditional stock pot is based on lots of gelatin-rich, flavorful bones and meat scraps, which of course you will not have in a low-fat kitchen. I do make good fish stock with fish trimmings and shrimp shells. But when

I make plain vegetable stock, it's usually pretty boring. You will need to decide whether it's worth your time, and whether you have the refrigerator space, to keep a stock pot going. Recipes for homemade stock are on pages 308–309, but really there are no set recipes. You start with boiling water, add the vegetables and scraps, and simmer as long as you like — at least an hour — and strain the broth. Don't add spices to the stock since you will be using it in another recipe.

Other Choices. You can use fat-free canned broth or consommé in any of my recipes that call for bouillon. If you want to experiment, you can use tomato or vegetable juice, bottled clam juice, or any of the other liquids listed in Chapter 8.

Stone Soup

The story goes that you put a stone in the pot, cover it with water, add the vegetables and cook it all over the fire. You serve the soup, take the stone out and save it to flavor the next batch.

> 1 onion, chopped
> 2 cloves garlic, minced
> 3 stalks celery, diced
> 6 cups bouillon (see page 187)
> 3 carrots, sliced
> 1 dried red pepper, crumbled
> 1 can (28 ounces) plum tomatoes, chopped
> 1 small head cabbage, cored and chopped
> 1 can white beans (cannellini), undrained
> 1/4 cup fresh basil leaves, chopped
> Freshly ground black pepper

Bring the onion, garlic, celery and 1/2 cup of the bouillon to a boil in a large pot. Simmer about 10 minutes, or until the vegetables are softened. Add the remaining bouillon, carrots, red pepper, tomatoes and cabbage; simmer 20 minutes or until the carrots are tender. Stir in the beans and basil leaves. Serve with ground black pepper to taste.

6 to 8 servings

Mulligatawny Soup

British colonists in India freely adapted the foods and spices they found there and brought their recipes back home. Mulligatawny is the Anglicized version of an Indian word for "pepper water."

2 onions, chopped
2 stalks celery, chopped
1 green pepper, chopped
6 cups bouillon (see page 187)
1 dried red pepper, crumbled
1 tablespoon turmeric
1 tablespoon ground coriander
2 carrots, chopped
2 red potatoes, diced
2 ripe tomatoes, chopped
Juice of 1 lemon
¼ cup cilantro leaves, chopped
Freshly ground black pepper

Bring the onions, celery, green pepper and ½ cup of the bouillon to a boil in a large pot. Simmer for 10 minutes. Add the remaining bouillon, seasonings, carrots and potatoes, and simmer 20 minutes, or until the vegetables are tender. Stir in the tomatoes, lemon juice and cilantro and simmer 5 minutes. Serve with ground black pepper to taste.

4 to 6 servings

Primo Minestrone

Minestrone means "big soup." I'm for that. You can double or triple this recipe and serve it to a crowd or freeze it for the weeks ahead.

> 2 onions, chopped
> 5 garlic cloves, minced
> 3 celery stalks, minced
> 1 green pepper, chopped
> 6 cups bouillon (see page 187)
> 1 can (28 ounces) plum tomatoes, chopped
> 1/2 cup dry red wine (optional)
> 1 tablespoon fresh oregano or 1 teaspoon dried
> 1 tablespoon fresh thyme or 1/2 teaspoon dried
> 1/2 teaspoon red pepper flakes or to taste
> 1/2 small head of cabbage, shredded
> 4 carrots, chopped
> 2 potatoes, diced
> 2 cans white beans, undrained, or 3 cups cooked
> 2 small zucchini, sliced
> 1/2 cup rotini, elbow macaroni or other small pasta
> 1/4 cup Italian parsley, chopped
> 1/4 cup fresh basil leaves, chopped
> Freshly ground black pepper

Bring the onion, garlic, celery, green pepper and 1/2 cup of the bouillon to a boil in a large pot. Simmer about 10 minutes, or until the vegetables are softened. Add the remaining bouillon, tomatoes, wine, spices, cabbage, carrots and potatoes, and simmer 20 minutes. Add the beans, zucchini, pasta, parsley and basil; cook an additional 8 to 10 minutes or until the pasta is tender. Serve with ground black pepper to taste.

6 to 8 servings

Harira

Harira is the traditional lemony soup used to break the Moslem fast of Ramadan. I think it's good for quieting hunger pangs anytime.

2 onions, chopped
3 stalks celery, diced
1 sweet red pepper, chopped
6 cups bouillon (see page 187)
1 teaspoon turmeric
1 teaspoon ground coriander
½ teaspoon cinnamon
¼ teaspoon cayenne or to taste
1 potato, chopped
2 carrots, chopped
1 can (28 ounces) tomatoes, chopped
1 zucchini, chopped
1 cup curly vermicelli or Chinese noodles, crumbled
1 can chick peas, undrained, or two cups cooked
¼ cup lemon juice
¼ cup Italian parsley, chopped
2 tablespoons mint leaves, chopped
Freshly ground black pepper

Bring the onion, celery, red pepper and ½ cup of the bouillon to a boil in a large pot. Simmer about 10 minutes to soften the vegetables. Add the remaining bouillon, spices, potato, carrots and tomatoes, and simmer 20 minutes. Stir in zucchini, noodles, chick peas and lemon juice, and cook 5 minutes. Serve garnished with the chopped parsley, mint and ground black pepper to taste.

6 to 8 servings

Garden Salad Soup

If you think lettuce is only for salad, try this unusual combination. Keep the cooking time short after you add the vegetables, so they don't lose their bright colors.

>2 onions, chopped
>4 cloves garlic, minced
>1 green pepper, chopped
>4 cups bouillon (see page 187)
>½ cup bulgur
>1 can (28 ounces) plum tomatoes, chopped
>1 dried red pepper, crumbled
>1 head romaine lettuce, shredded
>1 cup parsley, chopped
>1 cup fresh basil leaves, chopped
>1 cup baby limas (fresh or frozen)
>1 zucchini, diced
>1 cup peas (fresh or frozen)
>Freshly ground black pepper

Bring the onion, garlic, green pepper and ½ cup of the bouillon to a boil in a large pot. Simmer about 10 minutes to soften the vegetables. Add the remaining bouillon, bulgur, tomatoes and red pepper, and simmer 30 minutes. Add the lettuce, parsley, basil, limas, zucchini and peas, and cook 10 minutes, or until all of the vegetables are tender. Serve with freshly ground black pepper to taste.

4 to 6 servings

Pepperpot Soup

Whole peppercorns soften as they cook and impart a more subtle flavor than ground black pepper. I like to eat them, but you can scoop them out before serving the soup if you prefer.

>1 onion, chopped
>4 cloves garlic, minced
>2 stalks celery, chopped
>1 green pepper, chopped
>1 sweet red pepper, chopped
>6 cups bouillon (see page 187)

1 can (28 ounces) plum tomatoes, chopped
1 cup white wine (optional)
½ cup brown rice
1 tablespoon paprika
1 teaspoon red pepper flakes
10 whole peppercorns
¼ teaspoon cinnamon
¼ teaspoon ground cloves
½ cup Italian parsley, chopped

Combine all ingredients except the parsley in a large pot, bring to a boil and simmer 45 minutes, or until the rice is tender. Stir in the parsley and serve with freshly ground pepper to taste.

6 to 8 servings

Lebanese Soup

Coriander and artichoke hearts are the distinctive flavors here.

2 onions, chopped
4 cloves garlic, minced
6 cups bouillon (see page 187)
1 teaspoon ground coriander
Pinch cayenne or to taste
3 carrots, sliced
2 potatoes, diced
2 ripe tomatoes, chopped
2 packages (10 ounces each) frozen artichoke hearts
1 can chick peas, undrained, or 2 cups cooked
½ cup Italian parsley, chopped
Freshly ground black pepper
Lemon wedges

Bring the onion, garlic and ½ cup of the bouillon to a boil in a large pot. Simmer 10 minutes, or until the vegetables are softened. Add the remaining bouillon, spices, carrots and potatoes, and simmer 20 minutes. Stir in the tomatoes, artichoke hearts, chick peas and parsley, and simmer 2 to 3 minutes. Serve with lemon wedges and ground black pepper to taste.

4 to 6 servings

Pat's Double Chick Pea Soup

I like to cook up a huge batch of chick peas and keep them on hand for salads, snacks and great soups like this one.

8 cups bouillon (see page 187)
1 onion, chopped
4 cloves garlic, minced
1 ripe tomato, chopped
¼ cup chopped Italian parsley
1 bay leaf
1 dried red pepper, crumbled
4 cups cooked chick peas or 2 cans, undrained
1 pound fresh spinach, chopped
1 tablespoon vinegar
Freshly ground black pepper

Bring the bouillon, onion, garlic, tomato, parsley, bay leaf and red pepper to a boil in a large pot. Add 2 cups of the chick peas and simmer 30 minutes. Strain off most of the bouillon and set it aside. Puree the vegetables in a food mill or blender, then return them to the bouillon. Add the spinach and the remaining chick peas; simmer 10 minutes. Stir in the vinegar and serve with ground black pepper.

6 to 8 servings

Basque Stew

Those smart Basques know that fruit belongs in soup.

1 cup dried lima beans
1 onion, chopped
8 cups bouillon (see page 187)
1 cup brown rice or cracked wheat
1 cup pitted prunes, halved
1 cup dried apricots, halved
1 carrot, sliced
½ pound cabbage, chopped
¼ cup yellow split peas
1 teaspoon cinnamon
2 teaspoons sugar
1 tablespoon lemon juice

Soak the limas overnight. Drain and rinse. Bring the limas, onion and bouillon to a boil in a large pot and simmer 30 minutes. Add the brown rice or cracked wheat and cook 20 minutes. Add the remaining ingredients and simmer an additional 25 minutes, or until the beans and carrots are tender.

6 to 8 servings

Super Lentil Soup

How can you go wrong when you put lentils and brown rice in the same pot?

> 2 onions, chopped
> 4 garlic cloves, minced
> 3 stalks celery, chopped
> 8 cups bouillon (see page 187)
> 1 can (28 ounces) plum tomatoes, chopped
> 2 cups lentils
> 1 cup brown rice
> 4 carrots, grated
> 1 teaspoon marjoram
> 1 teaspoon thyme
> 1 bay leaf
> 1 or 2 dried red peppers, crumbled
> ½ cup Italian parsley, chopped
> 1 cup dry white wine (optional)
> Freshly ground pepper to taste

Combine all ingredients except the parsley, wine and black pepper in a large pot. Bring to a boil, reduce the heat and simmer, covered, 45 minutes, or until the lentils are tender. Stir in the parsley and wine, if desired. Serve with freshly ground black pepper.

6 to 8 servings

Green Lentil Potage

Cook the tiny green French lentils until they are tender but still slightly firm to the bite, not mushy.

1 onion, chopped
3 garlic cloves, minced
1 stalk celery, chopped
2 cups green lentils
8 cups bouillon (see page 187)
1 potato, diced
½ teaspoon ground coriander
½ teaspoon ground cumin
1 dried red pepper, crumbled
1 pound Swiss chard or spinach, chopped
Juice of 1 lemon
Freshly ground black pepper

Bring the onion, garlic, celery, lentils and bouillon to a boil in a large pot. Add the potato and spices; cover and simmer 20 minutes. Add the Swiss chard or spinach and cook 15 minutes more, or until the lentils are tender. Stir in the lemon juice and serve with ground black pepper to taste.

6 to 8 servings

Popeye's Special

Can you tell that I love lentils? Here they take on my favorite Italian seasonings plus tomatoes and spinach.

1 cup lentils
6 cups bouillon (see page 187)
2 onions, chopped
4 cloves garlic, minced
Pinch cayenne or to taste
½ teaspoon oregano
2 bay leaves
½ cup bulgur
¼ cup Italian parsley, chopped
1 can (28 ounces) plum tomatoes, chopped
1 pound spinach, torn in pieces
Freshly ground black pepper

Bring the lentils and bouillon to a boil in a large pot and cook 20 minutes, or until they are just barely tender. Add the onion, garlic, seasonings, bulgur, parsley and tomatoes, and simmer 20 to 30 minutes, or until the bulgur is tender. Remove the bay leaves. Put the spinach on top of the soup; cover the pot and simmer just until the spinach wilts, about 2 minutes. Stir the spinach into the soup and serve with ground black pepper to taste.

6 to 8 servings

Soupy Golden Dal

If you like the thick dal on page 147, you'll enjoy this thin version, too. It has the consistency of pea soup and could easily be made with split peas or any type of lentils. The orange soup looks nice (and tastes good) with a green salad and warm French bread. Or you can serve it as part of a buffet of Indian dishes.

> 1 cup orange lentils
> 4 carrots, chopped
> 1 onion, chopped
> 2 garlic cloves, minced
> 1 dried red pepper, crumbled
> 2 teaspoons curry powder
> 6 cups bouillon (see page 187)
> 1 teaspoon fresh tarragon leaves, chopped (optional)

Bring all of the ingredients except the tarragon to a boil in a large pot, and simmer 30 minutes, or until the lentils are tender. Mash or puree the soup in a blender or food mill. Reheat and add the chopped tarragon leaves.

4 to 6 servings

Spaghetti Squash Soup

The strands you pull from the cooked squash look like spaghetti, but they have a slightly crunchy texture.

> 1 spaghetti squash
> 6 cups bouillon (see page 187)
> 4 red onions, sliced
> 2 cloves garlic, minced
> ½ teaspoon red pepper flakes
> 2 tablespoons white vermouth (optional)
> 1 can chick peas, undrained, or 2 cups cooked
> ¼ cup Italian parsley, chopped
> Freshly ground black pepper

Preheat the oven to 350°F. Cut the squash in half and scoop out the seeds. Place the squash halves, cut side down, on a cookie sheet covered with aluminum foil; bake 1 hour. Meanwhile, bring the bouillon to a boil in a large pot and simmer the onion, garlic and red pepper flakes for 10 minutes. When the squash is cool enough to handle, run a fork over the flesh to separate it into spaghetti-like strands. Stir the squash, vermouth, chick peas and parsley into the bouillon, and simmer 15 to 20 minutes. Serve with ground black pepper to taste.

4 to 6 servings

Tangle Soup

Here's spaghetti squash in a soup again — this time with tomatoes. It can be mild or spicy; you call the shots by adding harissa at the end.

> 1 spaghetti squash
> 1 onion, chopped
> 1 garlic clove, minced
> ½ teaspoon red pepper flakes
> ¼ cup Italian parsley, chopped
> 4 cups bouillon (see page 187)
> 1 can (28 ounces) plum tomatoes, chopped
> Freshly ground black pepper
> Harissa (optional — page 307)

Preheat the oven to 350°F. Cut the squash in half and scoop out the seeds. Place the squash, cut side down, on a cookie sheet covered with aluminum foil and bake 1 hour. Meanwhile, simmer the remaining ingredients in a large covered soup pot. When the squash is cool enough to handle, remove the strands with a fork and add them to the soup. Serve with freshly ground pepper and stir in a small amount of harissa if desired.

4 to 6 servings

Barley Soup

When you cook a whole grain like barley right in the soup, it soaks up the flavors of the tomatoes, wine and seasonings.

> 1 onion, chopped
> 3 stalks celery, chopped
> 4 cloves garlic, minced
> 4 carrots, grated
> 8 cups bouillon (see page 187)
> 1 cup barley
> 1 teaspoon grated lemon rind
> 1 tablespoon fresh oregano or 1 teaspoon dried
> 10 black peppercorns
> ½ cup red wine (optional)
> ½ cup Italian parsley, chopped
> 2 ripe tomatoes, chopped
> 1 can (6 ounces) tomato paste
> ¼ cup fresh basil leaves, chopped
> Freshly ground black pepper

Bring the onion, celery, garlic, carrots and bouillon to a boil. Stir in the barley, lemon rind, oregano, peppercorns and wine. Simmer 2 hours, stirring frequently. Add the parsley, tomatoes and tomato paste and simmer another hour, adding additional water if needed. Stir in the basil leaves and serve with ground black pepper to taste.

6 to 8 servings

Roots and Barley

I was prejudiced against parsnips until I added one to this soup. Nutmeg makes a big difference.

    ½ cup pearl barley
    6 cups bouillon (see page 187)
    1 onion, chopped
    4 cloves garlic, minced
    2 carrots, sliced
    1 parsnip, peeled and diced
    1 small turnip, peeled and diced
    2 leeks, sliced (white part only)
    1 cup cabbage, shredded
    1 dried red pepper, crumbled
    1 teaspoon oregano
    ½ teaspoon nutmeg

Soak the barley in water overnight. Bring the bouillon, barley and the remaining ingredients to a boil in a large pot and simmer 45 minutes, or until all the vegetables are tender.

4 to 6 servings

Millet Soup

If you think millet is for the birds, taste it in this easy soup.

    1 onion, chopped
    3 stalks celery, chopped
    2 cloves garlic, minced
    6 cups bouillon (see page 187)
    1 dried red pepper, crumbled
    3 carrots, sliced
    ¼ cup shiitake mushrooms, sliced
    ¼ cup Italian parsley, chopped
    2 tablespoons fresh dill, chopped
    ½ teaspoon dried oregano or 1 tablespoon fresh
    ¼ teaspoon dried thyme or 1 teaspoon fresh
    ½ cup millet

Bring the onion, celery, garlic and ½ cup of the bouillon to a boil in a large pot and simmer 5 minutes. Add the remaining bouillon, red pepper, carrots, mushrooms, herbs and millet. Simmer 30 to 35 minutes, or until the millet is tender.

4 to 6 servings

Millet-Kraut Soup

I was skeptical about sauerkraut in a soup, but it works.

> 1/2 cup millet
> 2 onions, chopped
> 4 garlic cloves, minced
> 3 stalks celery, diced
> 1 dried red pepper, crumbled
> 8 cups bouillon (see page 187)
> 4 carrots, sliced
> 1 can (28 ounces) plum tomatoes, chopped
> 1 teaspoon caraway seed
> 1 pound sauerkraut, drained
> 2 potatoes, diced
> 1/2 pound spinach or other tender greens, torn in pieces
> Freshly ground black pepper

Toast the millet in a heavy frying pan over medium heat until golden, about 5 minutes; set aside. In a large pot, bring the onion, garlic, celery, red pepper and bouillon to a boil; simmer 10 minutes. Add the carrots, tomatoes, caraway seed and sauerkraut, and simmer 20 minutes. Add the potatoes and greens and simmer 20 minutes, or until potatoes are tender. Season with freshly ground black pepper to taste.

6 to 8 servings

Mother's Split Pea Soup

The perfect winter supper is a bowl of split pea soup, a chunk of crusty French bread and some fruit.

> 1 cup split peas
> 2 bay leaves
> 6 cups bouillon (see page 187)
> 2 onions, chopped
> 3 cloves garlic, minced
> 3 celery stalks, chopped
> 3 carrots, chopped
> 1 green pepper, chopped
> ¼ teaspoon red pepper flakes or to taste
> 1 tablespoon fresh thyme or ½ teaspoon dried
> 1 tablespoon fresh rosemary or ½ teaspoon dried
> ¼ cup fresh basil leaves, chopped
> Freshly ground black pepper

Bring the split peas, bay leaves and 5½ cups of the bouillon to a boil in a large pot and simmer until thick, about 45 minutes. Meanwhile, cook the onion, garlic, celery, carrots, green pepper, red pepper flakes, thyme and rosemary in the remaining ½ cup of bouillon for 15 to 20 minutes. Remove the bay leaves from the split peas and stir in the vegetables and fresh basil. Serve with ground black pepper to taste.

4 to 6 servings

One-Step Split Pea Soup

This split pea soup practically makes itself. Add some more spices if you like — curry powder would be nice.

> 2 cups dried split peas
> 8 cups bouillon (see page 187)
> 2 onions, chopped
> 4 carrots, chopped
> 3 stalks celery, chopped
> 1 bay leaf
> 1 tablespoon curry powder (optional)
> Freshly ground black pepper

Combine all the ingredients in a large pot, bring to a boil and simmer 45 to 60 minutes, stirring occasionally. Whisk to mash the peas, or if a very smooth soup is desired, puree it in a blender in batches. Serve with ground black pepper to taste.

6 to 8 servings

Split Pea Soup with Brown Rice

Spices are the key to this fragrant, thick soup. If you're not familiar with cardamom, give it a try in this recipe. Scandinavians bake with it; Indians use it in curries or just chew on the seeds like little candies.

> 1 cup split peas
> ½ cup brown rice
> 6 cups bouillon (see page 187)
> 3 onions, chopped
> 4 cloves garlic, minced
> 2 bay leaves
> 1 teaspoon ground cumin
> ½ teaspoon cinnamon
> ½ teaspoon ground cardamom
> Pinch cayenne or to taste
> 1 tablespoon lemon juice
> ½ cup Italian parsley, chopped
> Freshly ground black pepper

Bring the split peas, rice and 5½ cups of the bouillon to a boil in a large pot. Reduce the heat; cover and simmer 45 minutes, or until the peas and rice are both tender. Meanwhile, cook the onion, garlic and spices in the remaining ½ cup of bouillon for 15 minutes. When the peas and rice are done, stir in the onion mixture, lemon juice and parsley. Serve with ground black pepper to taste.

4 to 6 servings

Portuguese Bean Soup

This thick, savory soup is even better the second day. Serve it hot or cold.

1 pound dried lima beans
3 onions, chopped
6 cloves garlic, chopped
8 cups bouillon (see page 187)
4 medium potatoes, chopped
¼ teaspoon cayenne or to taste
1 bunch cilantro (about 1 cup of leaves), chopped

Soak the limas overnight. Drain and rinse. Bring the lima beans, onion, garlic and bouillon to a boil in a large pot and simmer until the beans are tender, 45 to 60 minutes. Remove about half of the beans and set aside; add the potatoes and cayenne. Cook 30 minutes, or until the potatoes are very tender. Add most of the cilantro, and puree the soup in batches in a food mill or blender. Return the soup to the pot and stir in the reserved beans. Garnish with additional chopped cilantro.

6 to 8 servings

Egyptian Bean Soup

Favas are big beans with a distinctive flavor. They aren't often available fresh in the United States, but they are very popular in Italy, France, Egypt and other countries around the Mediterranean. Canned fava beans work fine here.

2 onions, chopped
3 garlic cloves, minced
6 cups bouillon (see page 187)
2 teaspoons ground cumin
3 tablespoons sweet paprika
Pinch cayenne or to taste
1 bay leaf
3 carrots, chopped
1 can (28 ounces) plum tomatoes, chopped
2 cans fava beans, undrained, or 3 cups cooked
¼ cup Italian parsley, chopped
¼ cup lemon juice
Freshly ground black pepper

Bring the onion, garlic and ½ cup of the bouillon to a boil in a large pot and simmer about 10 minutes to soften the vegetables. Add the remaining bouillon, spices, carrots and tomatoes and simmer 20 minutes. Stir in the fava beans, parsley and lemon juice and serve with ground black pepper to taste.

6 to 8 servings

African Pea Soup

Fresh gingerroot and lots of spices spark this pretty puree studded with whole peas.

> 2 onions, chopped
> 3 cloves garlic, minced
> 1 teaspoon grated gingerroot
> ¼ teaspoon cayenne or to taste
> 1 teaspoon ground coriander
> 1 teaspoon ground cumin
> 1 teaspoon turmeric
> ¼ teaspoon ground cardamom
> ¼ teaspoon cinnamon
> 4 cups bouillon (see page 187)
> 1 sweet potato, diced
> 2 ripe tomatoes, chopped
> 3 cups fresh or frozen green peas
> Freshly ground black pepper

Bring the onion, garlic, seasonings and ½ cup of the bouillon to a boil in a large pot. Simmer 10 minutes, or until the vegetables are softened. Add the remaining bouillon, sweet potatoes and tomatoes and cook for 15 minutes. Add 2 cups of the peas, and cook 5 minutes. Puree the soup in batches in a blender; return to the pot and reheat. Add the remaining peas and cook until they are tender, about 5 minutes. Season with ground black pepper to taste.

4 to 6 servings

Succotash Chowder

Chili powder adds a southwestern touch to this chunky chowder.

> 1 onion, chopped
> 3 cups bouillon (see page 187)
> 2 red potatoes, diced
> 1 teaspoon chili powder
> 1 cup fresh or frozen lima beans
> 2 cups fresh or frozen corn
> 1 cup nonfat dry milk mixed in 1 cup cold water

Bring the onion and ½ cup of the bouillon to a boil in a large pot and simmer about 10 minutes. Add the remaining bouillon, potatoes and chili powder and bring to a boil; reduce the heat and simmer 15 minutes. Add the lima beans and cook 10 minutes, or until they are tender. Add the corn kernels and stir in the milk. Do not allow the soup to boil after adding the milk.

4 to 6 servings

Four-Root Soup

Don't bother to peel the carrots or celery root. A quick scrubbing with a plastic scouring pad works fine.

> 6 carrots, chopped
> 2 parsnips, chopped
> 1 large onion, chopped
> 1 celery root, chopped (or use 4 stalks of celery)
> 3 cups bouillon (see page 187)
> 3 cups skim milk
> ½ teaspoon nutmeg
> 1 tablespoon lemon juice
> Orange slices

Bring the vegetables and bouillon to a boil in a large pot and simmer 45 minutes. Puree the vegetables with a little of the liquid in a blender, in batches, and return to the soup pot. Add the milk, nutmeg and lemon juice. Reheat but do not boil. Serve garnished with orange slices and a little sprinkle of nutmeg.

6 to 8 servings

Tater-Leekie

Cock-a-leekie without the cock tastes just as good.

> 4 leeks, sliced (white part only)
> 2 potatoes, diced
> 1 dried red pepper, crumbled
> 6 cups bouillon (see page 187)
> 2 cups Italian parsley, chopped
> 1 cup dry white wine (optional)
> Freshly ground black pepper

Bring the leeks, potatoes, red pepper and bouillon to a boil in a large pot and simmer 30 minutes. Add the parsley and wine, if desired, and cook 5 more minutes. Puree in a blender in batches. Serve hot or cold with freshly ground black pepper.

4 to 6 servings

Fennel Soup

I don't know why fennel isn't a more popular vegetable; it should be a hit with anyone who likes licorice. Notice how nicely quick-cooking oatmeal thickens the soup.

> 1 large fennel bulb, sliced
> 1 large onion, chopped
> 8 cups bouillon (see page 187)
> 1/2 cup quick oatmeal
> 1 pound spinach, torn into pieces
> 1/4 cup fresh basil leaves, chopped
> Freshly ground black pepper to taste

Bring the fennel, onion and bouillon to a boil in a large pot and simmer for 20 to 25 minutes, or until the fennel is tender. Add the spinach and basil, then stir in the oatmeal; cook another 2 to 3 minutes. Do not allow the soup to boil after you add the oatmeal. Serve with ground black pepper to taste.

6 to 8 servings

German Embassy Soup

The ingredients are humble, but the finished soup is good enough for a state dinner.

> 1 onion, chopped
> 8 cups bouillon (see page 187)
> 2 potatoes, diced
> 2 cups sauerkraut
> 1 teaspoon whole black peppercorns
> 1 teaspoon mustard seed
> 1 bay leaf
> 1/2 teaspoon red pepper flakes
> 4 cups cooked small red beans or 2 cans kidney beans, undrained
> 1/2 cup Italian parsley, chopped
> Freshly ground black pepper

Bring the onion and 1/2 cup of the bouillon to a boil in a large pot and simmer until the onion is softened, 5 to 10 minutes. Add the remaining bouillon, potatoes, sauerkraut and seasonings, and simmer 20 minutes, or until the potatoes are tender. Stir in the beans and parsley and simmer 5 minutes. Serve with ground black pepper to taste.

6 to 8 servings

Carrot and Chick Pea Soup

Carrots always look the same, but some are nice and sweet while others are crunchy but rather tasteless. This soup is especially good when you get a batch of the sweet ones.

> 1 can chick peas, undrained
> 1 pound carrots, chopped
> 2 cloves garlic, chopped
> 1 onion, chopped
> 4 cups bouillon (see page 187)
> 1 tablespoon lemon juice
> Mint or cilantro leaves, chopped

Bring the vegetables and the bouillon to a boil in a large pot and simmer 20 minutes, or until the carrots are tender. Puree in a food mill or blender. Reheat, stir in lemon juice and serve garnished with the mint or cilantro leaves.

4 servings

Mushroom Farm Soup

I usually eat mushrooms raw or cook them just a short time, but the long cooking in this recipe yields an incredibly rich-tasting broth that is thickened with barley.

> 1 pound mushrooms, sliced
> 4 carrots, sliced
> 1 onion, chopped
> 3 stalks celery, sliced
> ½ cup barley
> 1 dried red pepper, crumbled
> 6 cups bouillon (see page 187)
> 1 pound kale, chopped, or 1 package frozen kale
> Freshly ground black pepper

Bring all the ingredients except the kale to a boil in a large pot and simmer 30 minutes. Add the kale and cook another 15 to 20 minutes, or until the kale is tender. (If using frozen kale, add 5 to 10 minutes before the end of the cooking time.) Serve with ground black pepper to taste.

4 to 6 servings

Caldo Verde (Green Soup)

Kale is my favorite green to use in this recipe, but you can substitute any leafy green or mixture of greens.

> 1 pound kale
> 3 onions, chopped
> 8 cups bouillon (see page 187)
> 1 teaspoon red pepper flakes
> 1 can white beans, undrained, or 2 cups cooked
> 2 potatoes, grated
> Freshly ground black pepper

Remove the center rib of each kale leaf and slice the greens into thin shreds. Combine the shredded kale, onion, bouillon and red pepper flakes in a large pot; bring to a boil and simmer 1 hour. Add the beans and potatoes and simmer ½ hour. Serve with ground black pepper to taste.

6 to 8 servings

Soups with Seafood

Soups that include fish and seafood are among the great treats of a low-fat diet. They can be thick and hearty or light and delicate. Nearly every region that has a shoreline has developed a traditional fish soupage Many of the classics — bouillabaisse, cioppino, Manhattan clam chowder, Maryland crab soup — suffer no loss of flavor when made without added fat.

Serving sizes for seafood soups are a little confusing. I recommend that you eat three or four 4-ounce portions of fish per week. The number of servings shown with each recipe is based on a reasonably sized bowl of soup, but a little seafood can flavor a lot of soup. Sometimes a soup that serves 8 will have only an ounce or two of seafood in each serving. That means you can have two bowls and count them as one "portion" of fish. On the other hand, the bounteous "fisherman's catch" soups — bouillabaisse, cioppino and the like — are so full of seafood that you will probably need to count a single bowlful as two "portions" of fish. Just remember to count about 4 ounces of the seafood itself as 1 serving when you tally your day's portions of low-fat/low-fiber foods.

Authentic Maryland Crab Soup

Authentic Maryland Crab Soup should be made with authentic Maryland blue crabs, but any crab meat will do. Tomatoes and corn are the hallmarks of the Real Thing. This is low-fat eating at its best.

> 2 onions, chopped
> 2 cloves garlic, minced
> 1 green pepper, chopped
> 3 stalks celery, chopped
> 6 cups fish stock or bouillon (see page 187)
> 2 cans (29 ounces each) tomato sauce
> 1 bay leaf

1 tablespoon fresh oregano or 1 teaspoon dried
2 dried red peppers, crumbled or to taste
2 potatoes, diced
4 carrots, sliced
2 cups fresh or frozen corn kernels
1 pound crab meat
½ cup Italian parsley, chopped
Freshly ground black pepper

Cook the onion, garlic, green pepper and celery in ½ cup of the stock to soften, 5 to 10 minutes. Add the remaining stock, tomato sauce, bay leaf, oregano, red peppers, potatoes and carrots and cook 20 minutes, or until the vegetables are tender. Stir in the corn, crabmeat and parsley and simmer 5 minutes. Serve with ground black pepper to taste.

8 to 10 servings

Banh Pho with Giant Prawns

Visits to a local Vietnamese restaurant inspired this recipe. You can find the fresh noodles in Asian grocery stores, or use dried ones from the international section of your supermarket. If you can't find giant prawns, use ½ pound of large shrimp.

6 cups fish stock (see page 187)
2 slices (¼ inch each) fresh gingerroot
2 cloves garlic, minced
3 green onions, sliced
1 small hot chile, sliced
1 tablespoon fish sauce
1 cup sliced bok choy or Chinese cabbage
Giant prawns (allow 1 to 2 per person)
Banh Pho (Vietnamese noodles), fresh or dried
1 cup bean sprouts
½ cup cilantro leaves, chopped

If dried noodles are used, soak in cold water to cover for 10 minutes. Bring the stock and seasonings to a boil and simmer 15 to 20 minutes. Remove the gingerroot and stir in the bok choy and prawns. Cook until the prawns are firm, about 3 to 5 minutes; remove them and stir in the noodles. Cook the noodles until they are *al dente* — 2 to 3 minutes for fresh, 6 to 8 for dried (check frequently so they do not overcook). Stir in the bean sprouts and cilantro and ladle into bowls; top each serving with 1 or 2 of the prawns.

4 to 6 servings

Thai Shrimp Soup

I love Thai food, and my favorite dishes are the soups. You can make this one even if you don't have galanga, lime leaves or lemon grass, but the authentic ingredients make the broth fragrant and special.

> 6 cups fish stock (see page 187)
> 2 stalks lemon grass, crushed (see page 314)
> 2 slices galanga (see page 314)
> 4 kaffir lime leaves (see page 314) or 1 teaspoon grated lime rind
> 4 cloves garlic, minced
> Stem and roots of one bunch of cilantro, chopped (reserve leaves)
> 1 small hot chile, sliced thin, or 1 dried red pepper, crumbled
> ½ pound shrimp
> 2 tablespoons fish sauce
> ¼ cup lime juice
> ¼ cup cilantro leaves, chopped
> Lime wedges

Bring the fish stock to a boil in a large pot; add the lemon grass, galanga, lime leaves, garlic, cilantro root and hot chile, and reduce the heat to simmer. Peel the shrimp and add the shrimp shells to the stock. Simmer the stock 20 to 30 minutes; strain and return it to the pot. Stir in the fish sauce and lime juice. Add the shrimp and cook 2 minutes. Top each bowl with cilantro leaves and serve with lime wedges.

4 to 6 servings

Bouillabaisse

Bouillabaisse is a true gourmet feast that can be made with whatever looks best in the seafood market. Remember that each "serving" is likely to have about 8 ounces, or two "portions," of seafood.

> 2 onions, sliced
> 2 leeks, sliced
> 6 cloves garlic, minced

3 cups fish stock or clam juice (see page 187)
1 can (28 ounces) plum tomatoes, chopped
2 carrots, chopped
6 potatoes, diced
2 bay leaves
½ teaspoon ground fennel
1 tablespoon grated orange rind
1 tablespoon fresh thyme or 1 teaspoon dried
2 tablespoons fresh marjoram or 2 teaspoons dried
½ teaspoon saffron threads
¼ teaspoon cayenne or to taste
3 pounds assorted fish and shellfish (fish fillets cut into chunks, shrimp,
   clams and mussels)
1 cup Italian parsley, chopped
½ cup fresh basil, chopped
Juice of 1 lemon
Freshly ground black pepper
French bread

Cook the onion, leeks and garlic in ½ cup of the stock to soften, about 5 minutes. Add the remaining stock, tomatoes, carrots, potatoes and seasonings, and simmer 20 minutes. Add the fish fillets, parsley, basil and lemon juice; simmer 5 minutes. Add scrubbed clams and/or mussels and cook 2 to 3 minutes, or until their shells start to open. Stir in the shrimp and cook 2 minutes more. Serve with ground black pepper to taste and crusty French bread.

6 to 8 servings
Count each serving as 2 portions of seafood.

Vietnamese Fisherman's Soup I

The Vietnamese know how to combine sweet and tart flavors for perfect low-fat soups. I love this so much that I want you to try two different versions.

> 4 cups fish stock (see page 187)
> 2 tablespoons lemon or lime juice
> 2 tablespoons sugar
> 2 large cloves roasted garlic (see page 313)
> 1 tablespoon fish sauce
> 1 onion, sliced
> 1 carrot, grated
> 1 can water chestnuts, sliced
> ¼ pound shrimp, peeled and sliced in half lengthwise
> ¼ pound haddock or any firm white fish fillets, cut in 1-inch chunks
> 1 ripe tomato, chopped
> 1 cup bean sprouts
> 2 tablespoons cilantro leaves, chopped
> 1 hot green chile, seeded and sliced

Bring the fish stock, lemon or lime juice, sugar, garlic and fish sauce to a boil. Add the onion, carrot and water chestnuts and simmer 15 minutes. Add the shrimp and fish; cook 2 to 3 minutes, or until the shrimp are pink and the fish is firm. Stir in the remaining ingredients and serve immediately.

4 to 6 servings

Vietnamese Fisherman's Soup II

Here's the second version — with pineapple.

> 4 cups fish stock (see page 187)
> 1 onion, chopped
> 1 garlic clove, minced
> 3 green onions, sliced
> 1 6-inch piece lemon grass, crushed (see page 314) or grated rind of one lemon
> ¼ teaspoon hot pepper sauce
> 2 star anise
> 2 tablespoons rice wine vinegar, lime or lemon juice

2 teaspoons sugar
1 carrot, grated
1 cup pineapple chunks, fresh or canned
1/2 pound flounder or other firm white fish fillets
1/2 pound shrimp, shelled
1 tablespoon soy sauce
1 ripe tomato, cut in wedges
1 cup bean sprouts
1/4 cup cilantro leaves, chopped

Heat the stock to boiling with the onion, garlic, lemon grass, pepper sauce, star anise, vinegar and sugar. Simmer 15 minutes; remove the lemon grass stalk and anise. Add the carrot, pineapple, fish and shrimp; cook 5 minutes, or until the fish is opaque. Add the soy sauce, tomato, bean sprouts and cilantro.

4 to 6 servings

Flounder Soup

Saffron tints the flounder and orzo with a golden glow.

1 onion, chopped
4 leeks, sliced
3 cloves garlic, minced
1 dried red pepper, crumbled
6 cups fish stock (see page 187)
1 can (28 ounces) plum tomatoes, chopped
1/2 teaspoon saffron threads
1/2 cup orzo (rice-shaped pasta)
1 pound flounder fillets, cut in 2-inch pieces
Freshly ground black pepper

Cook the onion, leeks, garlic and red pepper in stock for 10 minutes. Add the tomatoes and saffron and cook 20 minutes. Add the orzo and fish and cook until the pasta is *al dente*, about 10 minutes. Serve with ground black pepper to taste.

4 to 6 servings

Squid Soup

If you like squid, you'll love this soup. If you've never tried it, work up your courage, buy a box and follow the directions for preparing the strange-looking critters on page 178. Sometimes you can buy squid already thawed and cleaned at your fish market, but it's more expensive and you'll miss half the fun.

> 3-pound box of frozen squid or 1 ½ pounds thawed and cleaned
> 1 onion, chopped
> 4 cloves garlic, minced
> 1 green pepper, chopped
> 2 stalks celery, chopped
> 4 cups fish stock (see page 187)
> 1 can (29 ounces) tomato sauce
> 1 can (28 ounces) plum tomatoes, chopped
> 1 bay leaf
> 1 tablespoon fresh oregano or 1 teaspoon dried
> 2 dried red peppers, crumbled, or to taste
> 4 cups mixed vegetables, fresh or frozen
>   (cauliflower, carrots, Italian green beans, pearl onions)
> Cooked pasta shells or other small shapes
> Freshly ground black pepper

Clean the squid as shown in the directions on page 178, cut the body sacs into rings, and set aside. Cook the onion, garlic, green pepper and celery in ½ cup of the stock to soften, 5 to 10 minutes. Add the remaining stock, tomato sauce, tomatoes, bay leaf, oregano and red pepper and simmer 15 minutes. Add the mixed vegetables and cook 10 to 15 minutes, or until they are tender. Just before serving, stir in the squid; simmer 3 to 5 minutes. Do not overcook or the squid will toughen. Place a small amount of the pasta in each bowl, ladle in the soup and serve with ground black pepper to taste.

8 to 10 servings

Manhattan Clam Chowder with Limas

A good Manhattan chowder deserves to be full of beans.

>   1 onion, chopped
>   2 stalks celery, chopped
>   2 cups bottled clam juice
>   1 can (28 ounces) tomatoes, chopped
>   1 tablespoon fresh thyme or ½ teaspoon dried
>   Pinch cayenne or to taste
>   3 cups frozen lima beans
>   2 cans (7 ounces each) minced clams, undrained
>   ½ teaspoon Worcestershire sauce or to taste
>   ¼ cup Italian parsley, chopped
>   Freshly ground black pepper

Cook the onion, celery, clam juice and tomatoes with their juice for 10 minutes, or until the onion is softened. Add the thyme, cayenne and limas and cook 5 minutes; add the clams and Worcestershire. Stir in the parsley and serve; pass the pepper grinder.

4 servings

Chinese Scallop Soup

All my other recipes for scallops cook them for just a few minutes, but the effect here is entirely different. You cook them for a long time and then rub them between your fingers into little shreds. The taste and texture are unique.

>   6 cups fish stock (see page 187)
>   ½ pound sea scallops
>   3 slices gingerroot, each ¼-inch thick
>   2 tablespoons cornstarch
>   ¼ cup cold water
>   ¼ cup white wine
>   1 package (8 ounces) frozen sugar snap peas or ½ pound snow peas
>   6 scallions, sliced
>   Freshly ground black pepper

Bring the stock to a boil; add the scallops and gingerroot. Cover and simmer for 1 hour. Remove the scallops and ginger with a slotted spoon;

discard the ginger. Place the scallops in a colander; rinse with cold water and drain. Rub the scallops between your fingers to shred them into little pieces.

Mix the cornstarch and water in a cup. Bring the stock back to a boil and add the wine. Stir in the cornstarch mixture and simmer 5 minutes. Add the shredded scallops, peas and scallions and cook 2 to 3 minutes. Garnish each bowl with a few slices of the green scallion tops and add ground black pepper to taste.

4 to 6 servings

Scallop and Lemon Grass Soup

If I find fresh lemon grass in an Asian grocery store, I change my shopping list and make this soup.

> 4 cups fish stock, clam juice or bouillon (see page 187)
> ½ cup sliced green onions
> 1 garlic clove, minced
> 3 stalks fresh lemon grass, crushed (see page 314)
> 1 dried red pepper, crumbled
> 1 slice (¼ inch) gingerroot
> ½ pound scallops, quartered if large
> ½ cup Italian parsley, chopped

Simmer all ingredients except the scallops and parsley for 30 minutes. Strain the stock, discarding the vegetables. Reheat the stock to a simmer; add the scallops and parsley and cook 1 minute.

4 servings

Seafood Chowder

I haven't found any way to duplicate the sinful richness of the fat-laden New England chowders, but this one comes close.

> 6 cups fish stock or bouillon (see page 187)
> 1 cup bottled clam juice
> 1 pound shrimp
> 1 onion, chopped
> 3 stalks celery, diced
> 3 carrots, chopped

4 medium potatoes, peeled and diced
2 tablespoons fresh thyme or 1 teaspoon dried
Pinch cayenne or to taste
2 cans (7 ounces each) minced clams, undrained
1 pound crab meat or crab surimi
2 cups milk
2 tablespoons flour
1 teaspoon paprika

Bring the stock and clam juice to a boil; add the shrimp and cook 2 minutes. Remove the shrimp with a slotted spoon and set aside. Add the onion, celery, carrots, potatoes, thyme and cayenne to the stock and simmer 20 minutes, or until the potatoes are soft. Meanwhile, peel the shrimp and cut into 2 or 3 pieces. Stir the flour into ½ cup of the milk and set aside. Add the shrimp, clams and crab to the soup. Stir in the milk/flour mixture, the remaining milk and paprika. Cook 5 minutes; do not allow the soup to boil after you add the milk.

6 to 8 servings
Each serving counts as 2 portions of seafood.

Portuguese Seafood Stew

This is one of those wonderful seafood soup/stew recipes that can be made from any combination of low-fat fish or shellfish that appeals to you. Use whatever looks good or is on special at your fish market — you can't go wrong. Serve with a green salad and French bread.

1 large onion, chopped
3 cloves garlic, chopped
4 stalks celery, chopped
1 green pepper, chopped
6 cups fish stock or bouillon (see page 187)
1 can (28 ounces) plum tomatoes, chopped
3 dried red peppers, crumbled, or ¼ teaspoon cayenne or to taste
1 teaspoon oregano
2 cups water
1 pound medium shrimp
1 pound firm white fish fillets (flounder, halibut, orange roughy, perch)
1 pound mussels
4 red potatoes, cut into ½-inch cubes
1 pint oysters, undrained
½ cup cilantro leaves, chopped

Cook the onion, garlic, celery and pepper in 1 cup of the stock until soft. Add the remaining stock, tomatoes, pepper and oregano; bring to a boil and simmer, uncovered, for ½ hour.

Meanwhile, prepare the seafood. Bring the water to a boil, add the shrimp and cook just until they turn pink, about 2 minutes. Add the cooking water to the stew pot and set the shrimp aside to cool. Cut the fillets into 2-inch pieces. Rinse the mussels and throw out any that are open or broken; remove the beards and return the mussels to the refrigerator. Peel the shrimp and set aside.

Add the potatoes to the stew pot and continue cooking for 20 minutes, or until they are soft. Add more bouillon or water if needed — make the stew as soupy as you like. Then add the fish fillets, the oysters and the mussels and cook just until the mussel shells open (3 to 5 minutes). Stir in the shrimp and the cilantro.

8 to 10 servings
Each serving counts as 2 portions of seafood.

Cioppino

Cioppino is the Italian answer to bouillabaisse. You can use any combination of seafood in this basic recipe. Three jalapeño peppers make the soup quite spicy; if you are nervous about the heat, use cayenne pepper instead and add a pinch at a time, tasting as you go. The soup keeps well for several days; reheat it gently.

> 2 cups fish stock or bouillon (see page 187)
> 1 large onion, chopped
> 4 cloves garlic, chopped
> 4 stalks celery, chopped
> 1 large green pepper, chopped
> 3 jalapeño peppers, sliced, or cayenne to taste
> 2 cans (28 ounces each) plum tomatoes, chopped
> 2 tablespoons fresh oregano or 1 teaspoon dried
> 1 tablespoon fresh thyme or ½ teaspoon dried
> 1 bay leaf
> 12 cherrystone clams
> 1 pound shrimp, unshelled
> 1 pound bay scallops
> 1 pound cleaned squid, cut in rings or 1-inch squares

Bring the stock to a boil; add the onion, garlic, celery and peppers and simmer 10 minutes. Add the tomatoes and herbs, and simmer 20 minutes. Add the clams and simmer a few minutes, until their shells begin to open. Then stir in the shrimp, scallops and squid and simmer about 5 minutes more, until the shrimp shells are pink. Serve with warm French bread and a green salad.

8 to 10 servings
Each serving counts as 2 portions of seafood.

Golden Bowl

This soup contrasts beautifully with a crisp green salad.

1 large onion, chopped
4 leeks, chopped (include some of the green)
4 cloves garlic, chopped
6 cups fish stock or bouillon (see page 187)
2 cups bottled clam juice
1 can (6 ounces) tomato paste
1 teaspoon saffron threads
1 pound haddock or other lean white fish fillets, cut in 2-inch pieces
½ pound scallops
½ pound shrimp, peeled
½ cup Italian parsley, chopped, plus additional for garnish
¼ cup fresh basil leaves, chopped
Freshly ground black pepper

Cook the onion, leeks and garlic in 1 cup of the stock 10 minutes. Add the remaining stock, clam juice, tomato paste and saffron. Bring to a boil; reduce the heat and add the fish. Simmer gently 5 to 10 minutes, or until the fish is opaque. Add the scallops and shrimp and cook another 3 to 5 minutes, until the shrimp are pink and the scallops are firm. Stir in the parsley and basil. Ladle the soup into bowls, garnish with parsley and pass the pepper grinder.

6 to 8 servings

Thai Taste Noodles in Broth

In this and the next two soups, you can use any type of oriental noodle or even fettucine. Asian groceries have so many kinds of noodles, both fresh and dried, that it's fun to experiment.

> 8 ounces rice sticks (rice noodles)
> 6 cups fish stock or bouillon (see page 187)
> 1 bunch fresh cilantro
> 1 clove garlic, peeled and minced
> ¼-inch slice gingerroot
> ½ teaspoon crushed red pepper
> 1 stalk lemon grass (if available)
> 2 tablespoons oriental fish sauce (optional)
> 1 can (4 ounces) tiny cocktail shrimp
> Juice of ½ lime

Soak the rice sticks (flat rice noodles, about ¼ inch wide) in water to cover while you prepare the soup. Bring the stock to a boil in a large pot; add the stems and roots (if available) of the cilantro (save the leaves for later), garlic, ginger and pepper. If you can get fresh lemon grass, cut off the roots and slice the bottom 3 inches of the stalk into small pieces; add to the stock. Add the fish sauce if desired. Simmer 20 minutes. Strain and return the liquid to the pot; reheat to boiling. Add the noodles and cook 3 to 4 minutes, until the noodles are tender but still firm (al dente). Remove from the heat; add the shrimp, lime juice and the reserved cilantro leaves, coarsely chopped.

4 servings

Oriental Crab or Surimi Soup

You can use either real crab or surimi in this richly textured soup (see About Surimi on page 172). No one will be fooled by the brightly colored surimi, but it's inexpensive and quite tasty. Don't allow it to cook more than a few minutes.

> 8 ounces rice sticks (rice noodles)
> 8 cups fish stock or dashi (see page 187)
> 1 bunch scallions, sliced
> 2 cups Chinese cabbage, slivered

¼-inch slice gingerroot
1 dried hot pepper, crumbled
Juice of ½ lemon
½ pound crab meat or surimi (see page 172)
1 cup frozen corn, thawed
½ cup cilantro leaves, chopped

Soak the rice sticks in cold water while you prepare the soup. Bring the fish stock to a boil, add the scallions, Chinese cabbage, ginger and hot pepper. Simmer 15 to 20 minutes; remove the ginger and add the lemon juice. Return to a boil; add the noodles and cook until they are tender (about 5 minutes). Add the crab or surimi and corn. Ladle into bowls and top with the cilantro.

4 to 6 servings

Soba with Greens

Soba, the noodle made with buckwheat flour, is favored by the Japanese and should be more widely used here. Buckwheat is a very rich source of fiber. Imported foods don't have the same labeling requirements as foods made in the United States, so I don't know what percentage of the noodle flour is buckwheat, or the actual fiber content. I can only assume that it's higher than that of our pastas, which are made with refined wheat flour, or of other oriental noodles that are made with white rice flour.

8 ounces soba (Japanese buckwheat noodles)
Water
6 cups fish stock or dashi (see page 187)
½ pound chopped spinach or other tender greens
3 green onions, sliced
¼ pound surimi crab legs, cut in ½-inch pieces, or small peeled shrimp

Cook the soba in boiling water 5 to 7 minutes, or until firm but tender (*al dente*). Rinse in cold water and drain. Bring the stock to a boil; reduce the heat and stir in the greens. Simmer 3 minutes, then stir in the soba, green onions and seafood.

4 to 6 servings

Light Soups

The soups in this section are made with a single vegetable or combination of vegetables. Some have noodles or other starch. They do not contain beans or seafood, so you will need another source of protein.

A light soup served with a bean or seafood salad makes a perfect mid-day or evening meal. Several of these soups are delicious cold, so they are ideal for hot summer days.

Gazpacho

Gazpacho is my all-time favorite summer soup. I've included two recipes, but the truth is, you can combine the basic ingredients in any quantity you like and add your own personal touches with guaranteed success. Just make sure the tomatoes are really ripe; preferably they'll come from your own garden or a local produce stand.

> 2 medium cucumbers, peeled and chopped
> 8 ripe tomatoes, peeled and chopped
> 1 large onion, chopped
> 5 cloves garlic, peeled
> 1 green pepper, chopped
> 4 cups cubed pita or French bread (no crusts)
> 4 cups bouillon (see page 187)
> 1/4 cup red wine vinegar
> 1 teaspoon salt
> Freshly ground black pepper

Combine all the ingredients; puree in a blender and chill. If desired, garnish with additional chopped cucumber, onions or green peppers.

4 to 6 servings

Chunky Gazpacho

The preceding recipe blends the vegetables into a smooth puree; this one leaves them in small pieces. Try them both and decide which you prefer.

> 8 ripe tomatoes, peeled and chopped
> 2 cucumbers, peeled, seeded and chopped
> 1 onion, chopped
> 5 green onions, sliced
> 2 cloves garlic, minced
> 1 teaspoon horseradish
> 1 tablespoon fresh oregano or 1 teaspoon dried
> ¼ cup fresh basil leaves, chopped
> ¼ cup Italian parsley, chopped
> ½ teaspoon Worcestershire sauce
> Juice of 1 lemon
> 4 cups tomato juice
> ¼ teaspoon hot pepper sauce
> Freshly ground black pepper

Mix all the ingredients and refrigerate 4 hours or overnight. Serve with additional ground black pepper and hot pepper sauce to taste.

4 to 6 servings

Cold Sweet Red Pepper Soup

Those gorgeous big sweet red peppers in the produce section cry out for creative recipes. This one is easy and superb. It's also a good chance to try buttermilk, a cultured skim milk product with a taste similar to that of yogurt. It's a worthwhile addition to lots of summer soups. Check the label to make sure your buttermilk is fat free.

> 3 large sweet red peppers
> 4 leeks, sliced (white part only)
> 2 cups stock
> 2 cups buttermilk
> Freshly ground black pepper

Roast the peppers over a gas flame or broil until the skin is charred. Place in a paper bag and allow to cool. Peel the peppers, remove the stems and seeds and cut into chunks. Bring the stock to a boil; add the leeks and simmer 20 minutes. Add the peppers and simmer 20 minutes more. Cool; puree in a blender. Add buttermilk and freshly ground black pepper to taste. Serve chilled.

4 servings

Tomato Soup with Couscous

This simple soup can be as bland or as fiery as you like.

> 3 cups bouillon (see page 187)
> 1 small onion, chopped
> 1 can (28 ounces) plum tomatoes, chopped
> ½ teaspoon oregano
> Pinch cayenne or to taste
> ½ cup couscous
> Harissa (optional; see page 307)

Bring 2 cups of the bouillon, the onion, tomatoes, oregano and cayenne to a boil and simmer gently 20 minutes. Meanwhile, bring the remaining cup of the bouillon to a boil in a small pot. Stir in the couscous; cover and set aside for 10 minutes, or until the liquid is absorbed. Stir the couscous into the soup and serve. If you wish, pass a small dish of harissa with the soup and let diners stir in a tiny bit to get the amount of heat they prefer.

4 servings

Curried Broccoli Soup

This soup is equally appealing in summer or in the dead of winter. Orange slices set off the pale green, fragrant puree to perfection.

> 1 head broccoli
> 2 potatoes, unpeeled
> 2 cloves garlic
> 6 cups bouillon (see page 187)
> 1 teaspoon curry powder
> ½ teaspoon grated orange rind
> Orange slices

Chop the broccoli, potatoes and garlic. Simmer in the bouillon until the vegetables are soft, about 20 minutes. Add the curry powder and the orange rind; cook 5 more minutes. Puree in a blender and serve warm or chilled. Garnish with the orange slices.

4 to 6 servings

Creamy Yam Soup

Yams lend their bright color and smooth texture to a soup that will surprise you.

> 2 large yams
> 4 leeks, sliced (white part only)
> 4 ripe tomatoes, peeled, seeded and chopped
> 10 fresh basil leaves, chopped
> 4 cups bouillon (see page 187)
> Freshly ground black pepper

Bake or boil the yams until they are soft; peel and mash them. Meanwhile, simmer the leeks, tomatoes and basil in the bouillon 20 minutes. Puree the soup in batches in a blender. Return the soup to the pot and stir in the mashed yams. Serve with freshly ground black pepper to taste.

4 servings

The Zucchini Solution

When my patients or neighbors share the surplus squash from their gardens with me, I whip up a batch of this soup.

> 4 zucchini, chopped
> 1 onion, chopped
> 1 clove garlic, minced
> 2 teaspoons curry powder
> 2 tablespoons Dijon mustard
> 4 cups bouillon (see page 187)
> 1 cup nonfat yogurt or buttermilk
> 1 cup cooked brown rice

Simmer the zucchini, onion, garlic and seasonings in the bouillon 15 minutes. Puree the soup in batches in a blender. Stir in the yogurt or buttermilk and the brown rice. Serve warm or chilled.

4 to 6 servings

Squash Soup

Butternut squash is available all year, but somehow fall seems like the right time for this soup. I use it as a first course for Thanksgiving dinner.

> 2 butternut squash, peeled and cut into cubes
> 4 carrots, sliced
> 1 onion, sliced
> 6 cups bouillon (see page 187)
> 2 tablespoons brown sugar
> 2 tablespoons grated fresh gingerroot
> ½ teaspoon cinnamon
> ½ teaspoon mace
> Pinch cayenne or to taste
> Juice of 1 lemon

Combine all the ingredients except the lemon juice and cook 30 minutes, or until the squash is tender. Stir in the lemon juice and puree the soup in batches in a blender. Serve sprinkled with additional cinnamon, if desired.

6 to 8 servings

Soba with Shiitake Mushrooms

The woodsy flavor of shiitake mushrooms makes a rich broth. You can substitute regular mushrooms if you like.

> 10 dried shiitake mushroom caps
> 2 cups boiling water
> 3½ cups dashi or fish stock (see page 187)
> 5 tablespoons soy sauce
> ½ teaspoon red pepper flakes
> ½ cup sake (optional)
> 1 carrot, sliced thin
> 6 scallions, sliced
> 2 cups Chinese cabbage or bok choy, sliced
> 1 pound soba (Japanese buckwheat) noodles or other oriental noodles

Pour water over the mushroom caps and soak 20 minutes. Heat the stock, soy sauce, pepper flakes, sake, carrots, scallions and Chinese cabbage and cook 15 minutes. Add the mushroom soaking liquid to the pot; cut the mushroom caps into strips and add them to the broth. Meanwhile, cook the soba in boiling water 6 to 7 minutes or until *al dente*. (If using another variety of noodle, follow the package directions.) Drain the noodles and rinse them in cold water. Put a portion of noodles in each bowl and ladle in about a cup of the vegetables and broth.

4 to 6 servings

Hearty Salads with Grains and Beans

Salads that include beans and whole grains can be the main course, especially during warm weather. Serve them on a bed of lettuce leaves or use them to stuff pita bread for a satisfying sandwich.

Sometimes I make my own salad dressings, but I'm often in a hurry and the fat-free bottled dressings and mayonnaise are a big convenience. Be sure to read about them on page 230.

Snappy Lentil Salad

Lentils are not just for casseroles and soups — they make great salads, too! When you cook lentils for a salad, test them frequently so you don't overcook them. Take them off the heat when they are just barely tender and still a little chewy; rinse them with cold water to stop the cooking. For a special treat, use the tiny green French lentils.

1 cup lentils
3 cups bouillon (see page 187)
1 green pepper, chopped
1 sweet red pepper, chopped
1 jalapeño pepper, seeded and chopped (optional)
6 green onions, sliced
1 clove garlic, minced
1 tablespoon fresh marjoram or ½ teaspoon dried
1 teaspoon fresh thyme or ¼ teaspoon dried
Juice of 1 lemon
¼ cup Italian parsley, chopped
¼ cup nonfat Italian dressing
1 ripe tomato, chopped

Cook the lentils in the bouillon 30 minutes, or until tender but not mushy; drain. Mix the lentils with the remaining ingredients except the Italian dressing and tomato and chill. When ready to serve, stir in the dressing and tomato. Garnish with additional parsley if desired.

6 to 8 servings

About Fat-Free Mayonnaise and Salad Dressings

Many of my salad recipes use fat-free mayonnaise or bottled salad dressings. Some of the fat-free salad dressings are very tasty, while others are just plain awful. Manufacturers seem to be getting the message that lots of us want good fat-free dressings, because they keep putting out new ones. I keep trying them, and I recommend you do the same until you find three or four favorites.

Many of them are very sweet and make good dressing for cole slaw, but if you're looking for a substitute for oil and vinegar, you will want to search out an unsweetened, or at least less sweet, Italian dressing. I usually add a little extra vinegar or the juice of a lemon or lime to give the dressing more tartness. Stir in fresh herbs and spices to add your own personal touch.

Fat-free dressings and mayonnaise lose their consistency quickly once they have been mixed with other ingredients. Add them just before serving. If you expect to have leftovers, set aside part of the salad before you mix in the mayonnaise or dressing. Or you can pour off any excess liquid and add more dressing or mayonnaise on the second day.

Curried Bean and Rice Salad

Cooked brown rice is another good salad ingredient to keep on hand. When you cook the rice with turmeric and curry powder, the grains take on a golden tone that makes a beautiful salad.

> 1 cup brown rice
> 1 teaspoon curry powder
> 1/2 teaspoon cinnamon
> 1/2 teaspoon turmeric
> 2 1/2 cups bouillon (see page 187)
> 1 can kidney beans, drained, or 2 cups cooked
> 1 red onion, chopped

1 small green pepper, chopped
1 cucumber, chopped
1 cup nonfat yogurt
1 tablespoon lime juice
1 ripe tomato, chopped
¼ cup Italian parsley, chopped
Freshly ground black pepper

Cook the rice and spices in the bouillon until tender but not mushy, about 40 minutes. Combine in a bowl with the beans, onion, green pepper, cucumber, yogurt and lime juice. Serve garnished with the tomato and parsley, adding ground black pepper to taste.

6 to 8 servings

Black Bean Salad

Next to chick peas, black beans are my favorite bean for salads. Always rinse canned ones thoroughly so they don't muddy up the colors of the other ingredients.

2 cans black beans, rinsed and drained, or 3 cups cooked
1 red onion, chopped
1 clove garlic, minced
1 green pepper, chopped
1 sweet red pepper, chopped
¼ cup rice wine vinegar
1 teaspoon cumin
Pinch cayenne or to taste
¼ cup cilantro leaves, chopped
Freshly ground pepper to taste

Combine all the ingredients and chill at least 20 minutes.

4 servings

Southwestern Bean Salad

If you are timid about hot peppers, take it easy with the jalapeño — their heat varies. You can substitute a pinch of cayenne if you like.

>2 cups cooked brown rice
>1 can pinto, kidney or black beans, drained
>2 cups cooked corn kernels (fresh or frozen)
>1 sweet red pepper, chopped
>1 small onion, chopped
>½ cup vinegar
>¼ cup cilantro leaves, chopped
>1 minced jalapeño pepper or cayenne to taste
>1 teaspoon chili powder

Combine all the ingredients. This tastes even better if you let it stand, refrigerated or at room temperature, 1 hour before serving.

6 to 8 servings

Moroccan Melange

You can make excellent salads with cooked, chilled vegetables. This melange is equally good warm, at room temperature or cold.

>1 large eggplant, peeled and diced
>4 cloves garlic, minced
>2 teaspoons cumin
>2 teaspoons paprika
>2 teaspoons freshly ground black pepper
>1 teaspoon salt
>¼ teaspoon cayenne or to taste
>2 green peppers, chopped
>2 jalapeño peppers, chopped, or to taste
>2 zucchini, diced
>1 can small white beans, drained, or 2 cups cooked
>4 ripe tomatoes, peeled and chopped (or use canned plum tomatoes)
>4 tablespoons white vinegar
>Lettuce
>Pita bread (optional)

Cook the eggplant, garlic and spices in enough water to cover 30 minutes. Add the peppers, zucchini, beans and tomatoes and cook, mashing and stirring gently, until most of the liquid evaporates. Cool and stir in the vinegar. Serve at room temperature or chilled, with lettuce and toasted pita bread, if desired.

6 to 8 servings

Sunshine Salad

For some reason I like golden raisins better than the dark ones, even though they taste pretty much the same. Here they are paired with turmeric-tinted rice for a salad that almost glows. The dressing is particularly good.

> 2½ cups bouillon (see page 187)
> 1 cup brown rice
> ½ teaspoon turmeric
> ½ cup golden raisins
> 1 bunch green onions, chopped
> 1 green pepper, chopped
> 1 can (5 ounces) water chestnuts, rinsed and sliced
> ¼ pound bean sprouts
> ½ cup cilantro leaves, chopped
> Lettuce

> **Dressing**
> 1 cup orange juice
> 1 tablespoon lemon juice
> 4 tablespoons soy sauce
> 1 clove garlic, pressed
> 1 teaspoon grated fresh ginger
> ½ cup nonfat mayonnaise

Bring the bouillon to a boil; add the brown rice and turmeric and simmer, covered, until the rice is tender but not mushy, about 40 minutes; chill. Combine with the remaining salad ingredients. Combine the dressing ingredients and stir into the rice mixture. If you prepare the salad ahead of time, stir in the nonfat mayonnaise just before serving.

6 to 8 servings

Green Lentil Salad

Many people have never seen the tiny green lentils and will wonder about your secret ingredient. Cook them until they are just barely tender and still firm to the bite.

1 cup green lentils
4 cups bouillon (see page 187)
2 bay leaves
1 small onion, chopped
1 clove garlic, minced
2 carrots, diced
2 stalks celery, chopped
1 ripe tomato, chopped
1 tablespoon fresh oregano or marjoram or ½ teaspoon dried
1 teaspoon fresh thyme or ¼ teaspoon dried
2 tablespoons wine vinegar
Freshly ground black pepper to taste
Lettuce leaves

Bring the lentils and bouillon to a boil and simmer 15 to 20 minutes, or until the lentils are just tender, not mushy. Drain and cool. Mix with the remaining ingredients except the lettuce. Chill if desired; serve on lettuce leaves or use as a filling for toasted pita bread.

4 servings

Bulgur and Lentil Salad

Bulgur is the easiest grain for salads. You don't have to cook it — just soak it in hot water or bouillon. Both bulgur and lentils are bland by themselves, so add lots of spices.

6 cups bouillon (see page 187)
1 cup bulgur
1 cup lentils
1 red onion, chopped
4 scallions, sliced
2 cloves garlic, minced
1 tablespoon Dijon mustard
3 tablespoons wine vinegar
¼ teaspoon hot pepper sauce

> ½ teaspoon Worcestershire sauce
> 1 teaspoon oregano
> ½ teaspoon cumin
> 1 cup Italian parsley, chopped
> ½ cup fresh basil leaves, chopped

Bring the bouillon to a boil in a medium saucepan. Place the bulgur in a bowl, pour 2 cups of the bouillon over it and set aside. Add the lentils to the remaining broth and cook 30 minutes, or until tender. Drain, reserving ¼ cup of the liquid. Stir in the bulgur, onion and scallions. Mix the remaining ingredients with the ¼ cup of cooking liquid and toss with the salad.

6 to 8 servings

Tabbouleh

So good, your friends will think you bought it at a Lebanese deli.

> 1 cup bulgur
> 1 onion, chopped
> 6 green onions, sliced
> 2 cups Italian parsley, chopped
> ½ cup mint, chopped
> ¼ cup lemon juice
> 2 ripe tomatoes, chopped
> ¼ cup nonfat mayonnaise
> Lettuce

Place the bulgur in a bowl and cover it with cold water; allow it to soak 2 to 3 hours or until the bulgur is soft. Line a colander with cheesecloth or a dish towel and pour in the bulgur; squeeze out all the excess moisture. Return the bulgur to the bowl and mix in the remaining ingredients except the mayonnaise. Chill at least 2 hours. Stir in the mayonnaise just before serving. Serve on lettuce leaves.

Tex-Mex variation: Add 1 sweet red pepper, chopped; 2 jalapeño peppers, seeded and minced; and ½ cup cilantro leaves, chopped.

6 to 8 servings

Southern Three-Bean Salad

How many possible combinations of beans are there for three-bean salad? I'm still working on trying them all.

> 2 cups frozen lima beans
> 2 cups frozen black-eyed peas
> 1 can kidney beans, drained
> 2 carrots, cut in julienne strips
> 1/2 cup nonfat Italian dressing
> 1/4 cup lemon juice
> Pinch cayenne or to taste
> 1 tablespoon fresh oregano or 1 teaspoon dried
> Lettuce

Cook the limas and black-eyed peas according to package directions until just tender. Mix all the ingredients except the lettuce and chill. Serve on lettuce leaves.

6 to 8 servings

Four-Bean Salad

Who says I have to stop with three beans? By the way, fresh herbs make a big difference in salads. Oregano is easy to grow; see page 65.

> 2 cups fresh or frozen green beans, in 1-inch pieces
> 2 cups fresh or frozen lima beans
> 1 can kidney beans, drained
> 1 can chick peas, drained
> 1 red onion, chopped
> 2 ripe tomatoes, chopped
> 1/2 cup nonfat Italian dressing
> Pinch cayenne or to taste
> 1 tablespoon fresh oregano or 1 teaspoon dried
> Juice of 1 lemon

Cook the green beans and limas in a little water until crisp-tender. Mix with the other beans, onion and tomatoes. Combine the dressing, cayenne, oregano and lemon juice and toss into the bean mixture. Chill at least 30 minutes before serving.

6 to 8 servings

Corn-fetti Salad

Corn is overlooked as a salad vegetable, and I don't know why. You can just thaw frozen corn; there's no need to cook it. Or you can cut the kernels from leftover corn on the cob.

> 1 cup corn kernels (frozen or fresh)
> 1 can chick peas, drained, or 2 cups cooked
> 1 cup diced celery
> ½ cup chopped onion
> ½ cup chopped green pepper
> 2 tablespoons chopped pimento
> ¼ cup nonfat Italian dressing

Thaw the frozen corn or cook the fresh corn briefly in boiling water. Combine the corn with the remaining ingredients. Chill and serve.

4 servings

Springtime Salad

You can make this with frozen asparagus, but that first fresh asparagus of the year is cause for a special celebration.

> 2½ cups bouillon (see page 187)
> 1 cup brown rice
> 1 teaspoon turmeric
> 1 pound fresh asparagus
> 2 cups chopped ripe tomato or halved cherry tomatoes
> 1 yellow bell pepper, sliced
> ½ cup golden raisins
> ¼ cup wine vinegar
> Pinch cayenne or to taste
> ½ cup nonfat Italian dressing

Bring the bouillon to a boil, add the brown rice and turmeric and simmer, covered, until the rice is tender but not mushy, about 40 minutes; let cool. Slice the asparagus on the diagonal into ½-inch pieces and steam in a little boiling water until crisp-tender, about 6 minutes; rinse in cold water. Combine all the ingredients except the dressing and chill several hours. When ready to serve, stir in the salad dressing.

4 to 6 servings

Bean and Cabbage Slaw

Most of the creamy fat-free salad dressings are quite sweet and are good in coleslaw.

> 1 can red kidney beans, drained
> 1 can chick peas, drained
> ½ small head cabbage, slivered
> 1 small onion, chopped
> 1 small green pepper, chopped
> Peppercorn ranch or other creamy nonfat dressing

Combine the vegetables and chill. When ready to serve, stir in the dressing.

6 to 8 servings

Quinoa Salad

The small round grains of quinoa (pronounced *keen-wa*) give an interesting texture to this fruity salad. The grain has a mild, slightly nutty flavor that is greatly enhanced by the spices.

> 1 cup quinoa
> 2½ cups bouillon (see page 187)
> 1 stalk celery, diced
> 4 tangerines, peeled and sectioned, or 1 cup canned mandarin orange
>   sections
> ¼ cup golden raisins or currants
> 4 scallions, sliced
> ½ cup chopped green pepper
> Juice and grated rind of 1 lime
> ¼ teaspoon ground coriander
> ¼ teaspoon cinnamon
> ¼ teaspoon ground allspice
> ¼ teaspoon cumin
> Pinch cayenne or to taste
> Nonfat Italian dressing (optional)

Bring the quinoa and bouillon to a boil and simmer, covered, 15 minutes, or until the quinoa is tender but not mushy. Drain and place in a bowl. Mix in the remaining ingredients and serve at room temperature or chilled. If the salad seems a bit dry, add a little Italian dressing or more lime juice.

4 servings

Gabe's Favorite Potato Salad

I never peel potatoes for salads. The skins of the red ones are pretty in a salad and if you throw them away, you waste their fiber. Just scrub the potatoes with a plastic scouring pad.

> 6 red potatoes
> ½ cup chopped celery
> ¼ cup chopped onion
> ½ cup nonfat yogurt
> ¼ cup Dijon mustard
> 2 teaspoons celery seed
> ¼ cup fresh dill, snipped
> Freshly ground pepper to taste
> ½ cup nonfat mayonnaise

Boil the potatoes until just tender, about 20 minutes. Cool and dice. Combine with the remaining ingredients except the mayonnaise and chill at least 30 minutes. Mix in the mayonnaise just before serving.

4 to 6 servings

Dilly Potato-Pea Salad

Peas, potatoes and dill are natural springtime partners. If you can get them, use several red-skinned baby new potatoes, cut in quarters.

> 2 potatoes, diced
> 2 carrots, diced
> 1 onion, chopped
> 1 clove garlic, minced
> ½ cup bouillon (see page 187)
> 1 cup fresh or frozen peas
> 1 can chick peas, drained, or 2 cups cooked
> 2 tablespoons fresh dill
> Freshly ground black pepper
> 2 tablespoons red wine vinegar
> Nonfat Italian dressing

Cook the potato, carrots, onion and garlic in the bouillon 15 minutes or until just tender. Add the peas and cook an additional 2 minutes. Remove from the heat; stir in the chick peas, dill, pepper and vinegar, and chill. When ready to serve, stir in enough salad dressing to moisten.

4 servings

Honey Mustard Potato Salad

I may not have a Rolls-Royce, but I appreciate a good Dijon mustard in my potato salad.

> 4 red potatoes
> ½ cup chopped red onion
> 1 green pepper, chopped
> 2 stalks celery, chopped
> 1 tablespoon lemon juice
> 1 tablespoon honey
> 2 tablespoons Dijon mustard
> ½ cup nonfat mayonnaise

Cut the potatoes into ½-inch dice and cook them in boiling water until just tender, about 15 to 20 minutes. Drain the potatoes and combine them with the remaining ingredients except the mayonnaise; chill at least 30 minutes. Stir in the mayonnaise just before serving.

4 servings

Green Bean and Potato Salad

What would summer be without lots of potato salads? Here's one with green beans.

> 1 pound green beans
> 6 red potatoes
> 1 red onion, chopped
> 1 clove garlic, minced
> 2 tablespoons wine vinegar
> 1 tablespoon fresh oregano leaves or ½ teaspoon dried
> Freshly ground pepper to taste
> ½ cup nonfat mayonnaise

Cut the green beans in 1-inch pieces and steam until they are crisp-tender. Cut the potatoes into ½-inch cubes and cook them until they are just tender, about 15 to 20 minutes. Drain and toss the potatoes with the onions, garlic, vinegar, oregano and pepper and chill several hours. Stir in the mayonnaise just before serving.

4 to 6 servings

Spicy Potato Salad

This potato salad has an Indian accent.

> 6 red potatoes
> 1 red onion, chopped
> ¼ cup Italian parsley, chopped
> 1 cup nonfat plain yogurt
> 1 teaspoon caraway seed
> ½ teaspoon ground cumin
> ½ teaspoon ground coriander
> ¼ teaspoon cayenne pepper or to taste

Cut the potatoes into ½-inch dice and cook them in boiling water until just tender, about 15 to 20 minutes. Rinse the potatoes in cold water, drain them and combine with the remaining ingredients. Chill at least an hour before serving.

4 to 6 servings

Wild Rice Fruit Salad

Wild rice is one of my favorite salad grains. This recipe can easily be doubled or tripled for an impressive party dish.

> 3 cups bouillon (see page 187)
> 1 cup wild rice
> ½ cup golden raisins
> ½ cup chopped green pepper
> 1 cup red seedless grapes, halved
> 1 bunch green onions, sliced
> ¼ cup Italian parsley, chopped
> 2 tablespoons lemon juice
> 1 teaspoon curry powder
> ½ cup nonfat mayonnaise or enough to moisten rice
> Mint leaves for garnish (optional)

Bring the bouillon to a boil and add the wild rice; cover and simmer 50 to 60 minutes, or until the rice is tender. Drain and chill at least 15 minutes. Combine with the remaining ingredients and garnish with mint leaves if desired.

4 servings

Tri-Color Wild Rice Salad

When you see bright red, yellow and green peppers lined up in the produce department, you just have to create a salad that will do them justice. Here it is.

> 3 cups bouillon (see page 187)
> 1 cup wild rice
> 6 green onions, sliced
> 1 green pepper, chopped
> 1 sweet red pepper, chopped
> 1 sweet yellow pepper, chopped
> 2 tablespoons lime juice
> ½ teaspoon dry mustard
> ¼ cup nonfat Italian dressing
> Freshly ground black pepper

Bring the bouillon to a boil; add the wild rice, cover and simmer 50 to 60 minutes, or until the grains are tender. Drain and chill at least 15 minutes. Combine the wild rice, onions and peppers in a bowl. Stir the lime juice and mustard into the Italian dressing and mix into the salad. Serve with ground black pepper to taste.

4 to 6 servings

Wild Rice and Lentil Salad

Pickled jalapeños are not as hot as fresh ones, but they can still have quite a bite. You may want to start with one and taste as you go.

> 6 cups bouillon, divided (see page 187)
> 1 cup wild rice
> 1 cup lentils
> ½ cup sliced radishes

6 green onions, sliced
3 pickled jalapeño peppers, chopped, or to taste
2 cloves garlic, minced
4 tablespoons lime juice
2 tablespoons Dijon mustard
½ cup nonfat mayonnaise
½ cup Italian parsley, chopped

Bring 3 cups of the bouillon to a boil; add the wild rice and simmer, covered, until the rice is tender, about 50 to 60 minutes. Meanwhile, bring the remaining 3 cups of bouillon and the lentils to a boil and simmer until the lentils are just tender, about 20 minutes. Drain and cool. Combine the rice, lentils and the remaining ingredients except the mayonnaise and parsley and chill 30 minutes. Just before serving, stir in the mayonnaise and sprinkle with parsley.

4 to 6 servings

Kasha Salad

Buckwheat is the very best source of fiber, and it's a delicious salad grain to boot. Make kasha a frequent ingredient in your salads.

1 cup kasha (buckwheat groats)
2 cups bouillon (see page 187)
1 cup broccoli florets, steamed crisp-tender
1 cucumber, chopped
1 sweet yellow pepper, chopped
1 tablespoon fresh oregano or 1 teaspoon dried
¼ cup Italian parsley, chopped
¼ cup nonfat Italian dressing
¼ cup lemon juice

Bring the bouillon to a boil; stir in the kasha and simmer, covered, 15 minutes, or until the liquid is absorbed. Cool; mix in remaining ingredients and chill at least 30 minutes.

4 servings

Jewelled Couscous Salad

Regular couscous is fine for this sweet-and-spicy salad, but the whole-wheat variety has more fiber.

> *2 cups bouillon (see page 187)*
> *½ teaspoon ground ginger*
> *½ teaspoon turmeric*
> *½ teaspoon cinnamon*
> *Pinch cayenne or to taste*
> *1 cup whole wheat couscous*
> *½ cup golden raisins or currants*
> *½ cup chopped dates*
> *½ cup dried apricots, chopped*
> *1 cup chopped celery*
> *½ cup chopped carrots*
> *½ cup minced green onions*
> *¼ cup Italian parsley, chopped*
> *Juice of 2 lemons*
> *½ cup nonfat mayonnaise*
> *Lettuce leaves (optional)*

Bring the bouillon and spices to a boil in a large pot. Stir in the couscous and cook for 2 minutes. Remove from the heat, cover and let sit 15 minutes. Stir to fluff; add the remaining ingredients except the mayonnaise and chill. Stir in the mayonnaise and serve on a bed of lettuce, if desired.

6 to 8 servings

Quick Couscous Salad

Any dried fruits work well in this salad. You could stir in some fresh fruit, too, such as grapes or chopped apples.

> *2 cups bouillon (see page 187)*
> *1 cup couscous*
> *1 teaspoon curry powder*
> *½ teaspoon cinnamon*
> *6 green onions, sliced*
> *1 cup dried apples, chopped*
> *½ cup golden raisins*
> *¼ cup nonfat Italian dressing*

Bring the bouillon to a boil and stir in the couscous, curry powder and cinnamon. Cook, stirring, 2 minutes; remove from the heat and stir in the green onions, dried apples and raisins. Cover and let stand 15 minutes. Place in a bowl and toss with the dressing. Serve at room temperature or chilled.

4 to 6 servings

Stan's Pasta Fagioli Salad

In summertime, I keep containers of cooked grains or pasta in the refrigerator to add to salads on the spur of the moment.

> 1 can kidney beans, drained, or 2 cups cooked
> 1 cup cooked macaroni
> 2 ripe tomatoes, chopped
> 3 stalks celery, chopped
> 1 green pepper, chopped
> 1 clove garlic, minced
> 1 tablespoon fresh oregano or ½ teaspoon dried
> ½ cup nonfat Italian dressing
> Freshly ground black pepper to taste

Combine all the ingredients except the dressing and black pepper and chill at least 30 minutes. Stir in the dressing just before serving and pass the pepper grinder.

4 servings

Salads with Seafood

These main-dish salads make perfect summertime meals. Any leftovers will be appreciated at lunch the next day. See the note on fat-free mayonnaise and salad dressings on page 230.

The number of servings given with each recipe doesn't necessarily match with the portion sizes of fish and shellfish. That's because the salads have lots of other ingredients besides seafood. As you tally your 5 daily servings of low-fat/low-fiber foods and your 3 to 4 servings of fish per week, just remember that 4 ounces of seafood equals 1 portion.

Amy's Seafood-Barley Salad

This exceptional salad will be the highlight of a summer party. Or indulge yourself — make the whole recipe and have two or three days of great suppers and lunches. Divide it into meal-size portions and add the mayonnaise to each just before serving.

> 3 cups bouillon (see page 187)
> 1 cup pearl barley
> 1 cup bottled clam juice
> Juice of 1 lemon
> 1 clove garlic, minced
> 1 bay leaf
> ½ teaspoon oregano
> ½ pound shrimp
> ½ pound scallops
> ½ pound lobster surimi
> 1 green pepper, chopped
> 1 jalapeño pepper, seeded and minced (optional)
> 6 green onions, sliced
> 1 cucumber peeled, seeded and diced
> 6 radishes, chopped
> ½ cup fresh basil leaves, chopped
> 1 tablespoon Dijon mustard or 1 tablespoon curry powder (your choice)
> ½ cup nonfat mayonnaise
> Freshly ground black pepper

Bring the bouillon and barley to a boil and simmer 30 to 40 minutes, or until the barley is tender; drain. Bring the clam juice, lemon juice, garlic, bay leaf and oregano to a boil. Add the shrimp and cook 2 minutes; remove with a slotted spoon. Return the liquid to a boil and add the scallops; cook 2 minutes and remove with a slotted spoon. Continue to boil the liquid until ¼ cup remains; cool. Peel the shrimp. If the scallops are large, cut them into bite-size pieces. Combine the barley, seafood and remaining ingredients except the mayonnaise and chill at least 30 minutes. Just before serving, stir in mayonnaise and grind on black pepper to taste.

8 to 10 servings

Curried Shrimp Salad

Curry powder in fat-free mayonnaise turns just about any combination of ingredients into a delicious salad.

>   4 cups water
>   1 pound shrimp
>   1 cup golden raisins
>   5 green onions, sliced
>   ¼ cup Italian parsley, chopped
>   ½ cup nonfat mayonnaise
>   2 teaspoons curry powder
>   1 teaspoon grated gingerroot
>   Salt and freshly ground pepper to taste

Bring the water to a boil; add the shrimp and simmer 2 minutes, or until the shrimp are pink and firm. Drain (reserving the liquid for fish stock, if desired). Rinse the shrimp in cold water and peel; chill at least 30 minutes. Combine with the remaining ingredients.

4 servings

Crab with Cucumbers

This is a Japanese specialty.

>   2 cucumbers, sliced thin
>   1 tablespoon salt
>   2 cups crab meat or surimi (see page 172)
>   ¼ cup soy sauce
>   2 tablespoons rice wine vinegar
>   ¼ teaspoon sugar

Mix the cucumbers and salt; place in a colander and let drain 45 minutes. Rinse well and drain. Combine with the remaining ingredients.

4 servings

Tropical Shrimp Salad

This salad has it all: the visual appeal of the bright greens and oranges, the spicy and sweet contrasting tastes; and the varied textures of soft bananas and crunchy vegetables.

> 4 cups water
> 1 pound shrimp
> 1 cup chopped celery
> 1 cup chopped green pepper
> 1 cup carrots, slivered
> 1 pound spinach, torn in small pieces
> ½ cup cilantro leaves, chopped
> 3 teaspoons lime juice
> 1 teaspoon grated lime rind
> 1 teaspoon sugar
> 1 teaspoon cumin
> Pinch cayenne or to taste
> 4 bananas, sliced

Bring the water to a boil; add the shrimp and simmer 2 minutes, or until the shrimp are pink and firm. Drain (reserving the liquid for fish stock, if desired). Rinse the shrimp in cold water and peel. Combine with the remaining ingredients except the bananas; mix well and chill at least 30 minutes. Stir the bananas in gently just before serving.

4 servings

Fisherman's Bounty

Here's a full meal that's the summertime equivalent of cioppino or bouillabaisse. All it needs is a loaf of crusty French bread.

> 4 cups water
> 1 bay leaf
> ¼ cup vinegar
> 4 cloves garlic
> 1 pound shrimp
> ½ pound scallops
> ½ pound squid, cleaned and cut into rings
> 2 dozen small clams
> 1 sweet red pepper, roasted, peeled and chopped (see page 138)
> ½ cup lemon juice

2 teaspoons dry mustard
1/2 teaspoon salt
Pinch cayenne or to taste
1/2 cup nonfat mayonnaise
Lettuce leaves (optional)

Bring the water to a boil with the bay leaf, vinegar and one clove of garlic, cut in half. Add the shrimp and cook 2 minutes; remove from the water with a slotted spoon and set aside to cool. Add the scallops; cook 1 minute and remove. Add the squid rings; cook 1 minute and remove. Pour off all but 1/2 inch of the liquid. Add the clams and steam until their shells open; remove the clam meat from the shells. Peel the shrimp. Place all the seafood in a bowl; add the chopped red pepper and the remaining three cloves of garlic, minced. Mix 1/2 cup of the cooking liquid, the lemon juice, mustard, salt and cayenne. Pour over the seafood and refrigerate 3 to 4 hours or overnight. Stir in the mayonnaise and serve on lettuce if desired.

6 to 8 servings

Tart Fruits with Shrimp, Thai Style

This is an unusual and intriguing combination of sweet, tart and spicy flavors with an oriental flair. The fruits listed are one possible combination; vary to suit your preferences and take advantage of what's available. Most of the fruits should be tart or slightly underripe.

1/2 pound shrimp, cooked, shelled and halved lengthwise
1 grapefruit, peeled, sectioned and cut in bite-size pieces
1 firm mango, peeled and cubed
1 star fruit, sliced
Seeds of 1 pomegranate
1 cup seedless grapes, halved
1 fresh small hot chile, seeded and minced, or to taste
3 green onions, minced
1 tablespoon brown sugar
1 tablespoon fish sauce
Juice of 1 lime

Combine the shrimp and fruits in a bowl. Mix the brown sugar, fish sauce and lime juice until the sugar is dissolved; stir into the fruit mixture and chill at least 30 minutes.

4 servings

Your Choice Seafood Salad

You can choose any combination of shellfish you like, and season them to your own taste. I use all of the spices on the list to dress my salad, but you can combine whichever ones appeal to you.

> ½ cup crabmeat, surimi or cooked shrimp, cut in ½-inch pieces
> 1 ripe tomato, chopped
> 4 green onions, sliced
> Romaine or iceberg lettuce, torn in pieces (about 3 cups)
> ¼ cup nonfat Italian dressing
> Juice of 1 lemon or lime
> 1 tablespoon soy sauce
> One or more of the following:
>> ¼ teaspoon 5-spice powder
>> ¼ teaspoon dry mustard
>> 1 clove garlic, minced
>> ½ teaspoon fennel seed
>> ½ teaspoon grated gingerroot
>> Freshly ground black pepper to taste

Combine the seafood, tomato, onion and lettuce in a bowl. Mix the Italian dressing, juice, soy sauce and your choice of the seasonings; pour over the salad and toss.

4 servings

South-of-the Border Tuna Salad

If you get bored with plain tuna salad, try this zesty variation.

> 1 can (6 ounces) water-packed tuna, drained
> 1 can (15½ ounces) kidney beans, drained and rinsed
> 3 oranges, peeled, halved and sliced
> 4 green onions, sliced
> ¼ cup nonfat Italian dressing
> Juice and grated peel of 1 lime
> 2 tablespoons chopped cilantro
> ½ teaspoon chili powder
> 1 teaspoon cumin seed
> Freshly ground black pepper to taste
> Lettuce leaves (optional)

Combine the tuna, beans, oranges and onion in a bowl. Mix the Italian dressing, lime juice and peel, cilantro, chili powder, cumin and pepper; pour over the salad and toss. Serve on lettuce leaves if desired.

4 servings

Millet and Scallop Salad

Millet and seafood make an unusual salad that's festive enough for a party. You can easily double or triple the recipe.

> *½ cup millet*
> *1¾ cups bottled clam juice, fish stock or bouillon, divided (see page 187)*
> *1 lemon*
> *2 cloves garlic, minced*
> *1 small onion or 2 shallots, minced*
> *1 dried red pepper, crumbled*
> *½ pound scallops or crabmeat*
> *1 jar roasted red peppers, chopped*
> *2 cucumbers, peeled, seeded and diced*
> *1 tablespoon Dijon mustard*
> *½ teaspoon fresh thyme leaves or ¼ teaspoon dried*
> *½ teaspoon curry powder*
> *½ cup nonfat mayonnaise*
> *Paprika*
> *¼ cup Italian parsley, chopped*
> *Sliced tomatoes*

Toast the millet in a heavy frying pan over medium heat until golden, about 5 minutes. Add 1¼ cups of the clam juice, fish stock or bouillon plus the juice from ½ of the lemon and bring to a boil; reduce heat and simmer, covered, 20 minutes. Remove from the heat and let stand 10 minutes.

Meanwhile, bring the remaining ½ cup of clam juice or stock to a boil with the garlic, onion and dried red pepper; stir in the scallops and cook for 2 minutes, or just until firm. Remove the scallops with a slotted spoon; reduce the cooking liquid to ¼ cup. If the scallops are large, cut them into ½-inch pieces.

Combine the millet mixture, scallops, cooking liquid, juice from the other ½ lemon and the remaining ingredients except the mayonnaise; chill 30 minutes. Just before serving, stir in the mayonnaise and sprinkle with paprika and parsley. Serve on sliced tomatoes.

4 servings

Lobster Surimi Salad

If you really want to live it up, make this salad with fresh lobster.

> 1 pound lobster surimi, cut into small pieces
> 1 cup chopped celery
> 1 cup chopped radishes
> 1 cucumber, chopped
> 2 teaspoons curry powder
> 1 cup nonfat mayonnaise
> Lettuce leaves (optional)

Mix all the ingredients except the mayonnaise and chill. Just before serving, stir in the mayonnaise. Serve on lettuce leaves or as a filling for pita bread sandwiches.

4 servings

Light Salads

You don't need a recipe for a great tossed salad. If you keep plenty of salad vegetables on hand — fresh lettuce, tomatoes, peppers, green onions, and all the rest — you can always put together a salad on a moment's notice. Fruit salads are easy, too; just combine a few varieties you like, and mix in nonfat mayonnaise or sprinkle on a little lemon juice.

You can make your own dressing or choose from the many fat-free dressings that are now available in supermarkets. Be sure to read the labels: lots of "lite" dressings still have 2 or more grams of fat per serving. You want the ones that say 0 grams of fat.

The recipes in this section are some particularly good light salads that I enjoy. Use them to spark your imagination for other combinations. Serve them with a hearty soup or casserole to make a whole meal.

Salad Starter

Some salad vegetables will keep for several days, while others wilt quickly and should be cut up just before you use them. You can prepare a large quantity of salad-starter vegetables and refrigerate them, ready to use as is or to combine at the last minute with other vegetables, such as lettuce, mushrooms, tomatoes, cucumbers, bean sprouts or green peppers, for a delicious tossed salad. They're also good for munching as a quick snack.

Choose any or all of the following:
  Raw cauliflower, broken in florets
  Raw broccoli, broken in florets
  Sliced carrots
  Sliced or chopped celery
  Sliced radishes
  Sliced green onions
  Canned or cooked chick peas, drained
  Cabbage, slivered
  Bok choy or Chinese cabbage, slivered

Combine the vegetables in a large container with a tight seal. Use some for today's salad, and store the rest for use over the next several days.

Mediterranean Salad

Basil, tomatoes and yogurt make an irresistible combination for a warm summer day.

  4 ripe tomatoes, diced
  2 cucumbers, peeled, seeded and diced
  1 onion, chopped
  2 cloves garlic, minced
  ½ cup nonfat yogurt
  1 tablespoon lemon juice
  ¼ cup fresh basil leaves, chopped

Combine all the ingredients and chill at least 20 minutes.

4 servings

Tomato, Cucumber and Mint Salad

Mint adds a cool, refreshing note to vine-ripened tomatoes and cucumbers. If you'd like to grow a patch of mint in your yard, see page 65.

  ½ cup tarragon vinegar
  ½ cup lemon juice
  ¼ cup sugar
  ¼ teaspoon salt

Freshly ground black pepper to taste
½ cup chopped mint
6 ripe tomatoes, sliced
3 cucumbers, sliced
Romaine lettuce
Mint leaves for garnish

Combine the vinegar, lemon juice, sugar, salt, pepper and mint; mix into the tomatoes and cucumbers and marinate at least 1 hour. Line a bowl with romaine leaves, place the tomatoes and cucumbers in the middle and garnish with additional mint leaves.

4 servings

Tomatoes with Pepper Salsa

A spicy salsa makes a great salad dressing.

1 green pepper, chopped fine
6 green onions, minced
1 clove garlic, minced
2 tablespoons cilantro leaves, chopped
1 jalapeño pepper, minced, or to taste
½ teaspoon ground cumin
1 tablespoon vinegar
4 very ripe tomatoes
2 cups bean sprouts

Combine all the ingredients except the tomatoes and sprouts; marinate 4 hours or overnight. Slice the tomatoes and arrange on a bed of sprouts; top with the salsa.

4 servings

Tomatoes and Basil

This is a summertime staple in my house. Use vine-ripened tomatoes from your garden or a local produce stand.

Sliced tomatoes
Chopped fresh basil leaves
Rice wine vinegar
Freshly ground black pepper to taste

Combine the ingredients in any quantity you wish.

Tomato, Cucumber and Onion Salad

Here's another simple tomato combination that's best with vine-ripened tomatoes and a big, sweet red onion.

4 tomatoes, sliced
2 cucumbers, sliced
1 red onion, chopped
¼ cup fresh basil leaves, chopped
¼ cup nonfat Italian dressing
Freshly ground black pepper

Combine all the ingredients and serve with ground pepper to taste.

4 servings

Super-Easy Coleslaw

Caraway seeds lift this coleslaw out of the ordinary. With this and the next two slaw recipes, you can make a large batch by doubling or tripling the recipe and combining everything but the mayonnaise. Stir a little mayonnaise into a meal-size portion just before serving.

½ head cabbage, slivered
4 carrots, grated
2 teaspoons caraway seed
¼ cup cider vinegar
¼ cup nonfat mayonnaise

Combine all the ingredients.

4 servings

Hawaiian Slaw

½ head cabbage, shredded
3 carrots, grated
1 cup canned crushed pineapple, drained
¼ cup rice wine vinegar
1 teaspoon grated gingerroot
1 teaspoon fennel seed
¼ cup nonfat mayonnaise

Combine the cabbage, carrots, pineapple, vinegar, gingerroot and fennel; chill. Stir in the mayonnaise just before serving.

4 servings

Red Slaw

½ cup chopped red cabbage
1 cup bean sprouts
3 stalks celery, diced (use tender inner stalks)
¼ cup rice vinegar
¼ cup nonfat mayonnaise or creamy Italian dressing

Combine all the ingredients.

4 servings

Gazpacho Salad Mold

A molded salad takes a little advance preparation, but the results are worth it. A fancy mold and some basil or mint leaves for garnish make it pretty enough for a party.

1 cucumber, peeled, seeded and chopped
1 onion, chopped
1 green pepper, chopped
2 cloves garlic, minced
1 tablespoon lemon juice
¼ teaspoon hot pepper sauce
½ teaspoon dried oregano

1 can (16 ounces) tomatoes
2 envelopes plain gelatin
1¼ cups spicy tomato or vegetable juice

Combine the fresh vegetables and seasonings in a bowl. Puree the tomatoes and 1 cup of the vegetable mixture in a blender. Soften the
gelatin in ¼ cup of the tomato juice; stir into the remaining juice until
the gelatin is dissolved. Combine the juice and the puree and chill until
thickened. Stir in the remaining vegetables; transfer to a mold and chill
until firm. Unmold on lettuce and serve.

4 servings

Artichoke Salad

Preparing fresh artichokes is a little time consuming, but they are delicious. If you are in a hurry, the frozen ones make an acceptable substitute.

4 fresh artichokes or 10 ounces frozen artichoke hearts
4 green onions, sliced
8 mushrooms, sliced
½ cucumber, diced
1 cup nonfat yogurt
1 tablespoon lemon juice
Freshly ground black pepper to taste

If you are using fresh artichokes, cook them in boiling water until you can
pierce the bottom easily with a fork (about 30 minutes); drain and cool.
Cut the stems off about ¼ inch from the base and remove all the leaves.
Scoop out the "choke" (the inner thistles) with a spoon. Cut the artichoke bottoms into eighths and chill.

If using frozen artichoke hearts, cook them according to the directions
on the package and chill.

When ready to serve, combine the artichokes with the remaining
ingredients.

4 to 6 servings

Asian Salad

Look for seasoned rice vinegar and chili-garlic paste in the oriental section of the supermarket or in a neighborhood Asian grocery. Asian groceries are wonderful sources of interesting salad ingredients.

½ head bok choy, sliced thin
3 carrots, grated
4 green onions, sliced
1 cup bean sprouts
½ cup cilantro leaves, chopped

Dressing
¼ cup seasoned rice vinegar
½ teaspoon chili-garlic paste or to taste

Mix the vegetables in a bowl and toss with the salad dressing.

4 servings

Spinach Salad

If you think spinach salad has to have fat-laden bacon and hard-boiled eggs, try my version with tangerine sections. I like it even better.

1 pound spinach, torn in pieces
4 tangerines, peeled and sectioned, or 1 cup canned mandarin orange
  sections
1 small onion, chopped
4 ounces mushrooms, sliced

Dressing
¼ cup nonfat Italian dressing
½ teaspoon dry mustard
½ teaspoon celery seed
Freshly ground black pepper to taste

Combine the salad ingredients and toss with the dressing.

4 servings

Eggplant Salad

Roasted eggplant has a smokey taste that's just right for salads. Don't worry if you don't remove all the skin; some charred bits won't hurt the taste or the appearance.

> 1 medium eggplant
> 1 large ripe tomato, chopped
> 1 green pepper, chopped
> 1 medium onion, chopped
> 2 cloves garlic, minced
> Nonfat Italian dressing
> 2 tablespoons red wine vinegar
> 1 tablespoon fresh oregano leaves or 1 teaspoon dried

Roast the eggplant over a gas flame, under a broiler or on a charcoal grill until the skin is charred and the flesh is soft, about 10 minutes. Cool it and rub the skin off with damp paper towels. Chop the pulp and mix it with the remaining ingredients; chill.

4 to 6 servings

Kohlrabi Salad

Kohlrabi is in the same family as cabbage, broccoli and cauliflower. It looks like a green apple with branches sticking out of it and tastes a lot like its cousins. Peel off the slightly tough skin and enjoy its crispy interior.

> 6 kohlrabi, peeled and cut into matchstick strips
> 2 onions, sliced
> 1/2 cup wine vinegar
> 1/4 cup sugar
> 1/2 teaspoon grated gingerroot
> 1 tablespoon fresh marjoram leaves
> 1/2 teaspoon red pepper flakes
> Salt and freshly ground pepper to taste

Combine all the ingredients and chill at least 2 hours before serving.

4 to 6 servings

Daikon Slaw

Daikon is a very mild, large white radish that is popular in Japan and other Asian countries but is still treated as a specialty vegetable here. I think it's worth seeking out. If you can't find it, you might substitute a small quantity of diced regular radishes. To make the salad especially attractive, use the fine blade of a mandoline (see page 265) or a food processor to shred the daikon and carrots.

> 1 medium head bok choy, shredded
> 1 cup grated daikon (white radish)
> 1 cup grated carrots
> 1 cup bean sprouts
> 6 green onions, sliced
> ¼ cup cilantro leaves, chopped
> ¼ cup rice vinegar

Combine all the ingredients.

6 to 8 servings

Waldorf Salad

Waldorf salad is a favorite of children and adults alike, and it loses nothing in the translation to this low-fat version.

> 2 red apples, cored and diced
> 2 green apples, cored and diced
> 2 tablespoons lemon juice
> 1 cup chopped celery
> 1 cup chopped raisins (or use ½ cup raisins and ½ cup dates)
> ¼ cup orange juice
> ½ cup nonfat mayonnaise

Toss the apples in the lemon juice. Mix with the remaining ingredients except the mayonnaise; cover and chill at least 30 minutes. Stir in the mayonnaise just before serving.

4 to 6 servings

Pomegranate and Banana Salad

It takes some work to extract the red promegranate seeds from the white membrane of the fruit, but they make such a pretty addition to a salad that it's worth the effort.

>   1 pomegranate
>   4 firm bananas
>   ¼ cup lime juice
>   2 tablespoons brown sugar

Quarter the pomegranate and remove the juicy seeds. Peel and slice the bananas. Combine the lime juice and brown sugar, and mix with the pomegranate seeds and bananas.

4 servings

Curried Fruit Salad

Knowing how much I love the flavor of curry, you shouldn't be surprised to see it in a fruit salad. Needless to say, you can make this treat with any fruits you like.

>   1 cup seedless grapes, halved
>   2 tangerines, peeled and sectild
>   2 bananas, sliced
>   1 tart apple, cored and chopped
>   1 stalk celery, chopped
>   ½ cup golden raisins
>   2 tablespoons lime juice
>   1 teaspoon curry powder
>   ½ cup nonfat mayonnaise
>   Romaine lettuce leaves, torn in pieces (optional)

Combine all the ingredients and serve on romaine leaves if desired. If you wish to prepare the fruits in advance, sprinkle them with the lime juice and chill. Mix the curry powder into the mayonnaise and stir in just before serving.

4 to 6 servings

Side Dishes with Grains and Starchy Vegetables

A ny of the whole grains can be cooked by themselves and served as a side dish. This section gives basic instructions for preparing whole grains and then offers a variety of ways to season them and combine them with other ingredients. Recipes for potatoes and sweet potatoes are included in this section, too.

Many of my recipes are adapted from the traditional side dishes of ethnic cuisines. You can serve any of them with broiled or steamed fish, bean dishes, or as part of a festive meal with several courses.

Basic Instructions for Cooking Whole Grains

The following recipes are for cooking grains on the stovetop. I highly recommend cooking brown rice and most of the other whole grains in an electric vegetable steamer or rice cooker (see page 264). They always come out perfectly and never stick to the bottom of the pot! Consult the instruction booklet that comes with your appliance for the ratio of liquid to dry grains and cooking times. Make lots; leftovers store well in your refrigerator and can be reheated in the microwave or used in salads.

Basic Brown Rice

1 cup brown rice
2½ cups bouillon (see page 187)

Bring the bouillon to a boil; stir in the brown rice and return to boiling. Reduce the heat, cover the pot and simmer 40 minutes, or until the rice is tender and the liquid is absorbed. Don't overcook brown rice; it tastes best when the grains are still separate and slightly firm.

About 2 cups

Basic Wild Rice

Directions on boxes of wild rice always instruct you to wash the rice and pick out any foreign objects, but I must admit I never do and I haven't suffered any ill consequences yet.

>   1 cup wild rice
>   3 cups bouillon (see page 187)

Bring the bouillon to a boil; stir in the wild rice and return to boiling. Reduce the heat, cover the pot and simmer 50 to 60 minutes, or until the rice is tender and most of the liquid is absorbed. Drain off any excess liquid. Don't overcook; wild rice should definitely be chewy and not mushy.

About 3 cups

Basic Kasha (Buckwheat Groats)

>   1 cup kasha
>   2 cups bouillon (see page 187)

Bring the bouillon to a boil; stir in the kasha and return to boiling. Reduce the heat, cover the pot and simmer 15 minutes, or until the kasha is tender and the liquid is absorbed.

If you wish, you can toast the kasha in a dry frying pan before you cook it. Just place the pan on a medium-hot burner, add the kasha and stir constantly 3 to 5 minutes. I usually skip this step, but try it both ways and see which you prefer.

About 2 cups

Basic Barley

>   1 cup pearl barley
>   3 cups bouillon (see page 187)

Bring the bouillon to a boil; stir in the barley and return to boiling. Reduce the heat, cover the pot and simmer 30 to 40 minutes, or until the barley is tender and most of the liquid is absorbed. Drain off excess liquid if necessary.

About 3 cups

Basic Millet

1 cup millet
2 cups bouillon (see page 187)

Bring the bouillon to a boil; stir in the millet and return to boiling. Reduce the heat, cover and simmer 20 minutes, or until the liquid is absorbed. The millet should be tender but not mushy. Remove the pot

---

Low-Fat Kitchen Equipment

Low-fat cooking doesn't require any special equipment. This is a list of some items that are indispensable in my kitchen.

Blender. I use a blender frequently for pureeing soups or sauces. You can also make a delicious "California Smoothie" by whirling a banana or two and any other fruits you have on hand in the blender with a cup of fruit juice.

Colander or large strainer. Good for draining steamed vegetables, noodles and pasta, and essential for making yogurt cheese.

Electric steamer or rice cooker. These wonderful countertop appliances are a boon for the fat-free cook. They make cooking whole grains a cinch and let you steam vegetables to perfection. If you get one with a fairly large rice basket, you can make enough whole grains to have leftovers for salads.

Food mill. This forerunner of the food processor looks like a strainer with a crank in the middle. It makes short work of pureeing soups, vegetables or fruits and is the easiest way to remove the skins and seeds from tomatoes.

Food processor. I do most of my vegetable chopping, slicing and shredding by hand, but a food processor is nice, especially if you are making large quantities. A tiny (1-cup) food processor is useful for chopping herbs or onions.

Garlic press. This makes preparing garlic a snap. You don't even have to peel the cloves. The old-fashioned, simple garlic press is best; it has a small, round receptacle and tiny holes. Don't bother with the "self-cleaning" ones; their holes are too large to be effective.

Knives. A couple of really good, sharp knives make cutting up all those fruits and vegetables a pleasure.

---

from the heat and let it stand, covered, 10 minutes. Fluff with a fork and serve.

Like kasha, millet can be toasted before cooking if you wish. Place a dry frying pan on a medium-hot burner, add the millet and stir 2 to 3 minutes, or until the grains begin to brown lightly and pop. Remove from the heat and add to the boiling bouillon.

About 3 cups

Mandoline and graters. A mandoline is a hand-held shredder with blades that cut anything from matchsticks to tiny threads. I bought mine in an Asian grocery store, but they are also available in kitchen supply stores. Shredded carrots and other "hard" vegetables look pretty in a salad or as a garnish. Graters are quicker and are heavily used in my kitchen.

Microwave oven. Almost all of the recipes for vegetables, grains and beans in this book could be prepared in a microwave. My personal preference is to cook on the stovetop and use the microwave for thawing frozen dishes and reheating leftovers.

Pepper grinder. I make my pitch for freshly ground pepper over and over again. For flavor and fragrance, there's just no comparison between grinding your own and buying it preground. Your pepper grinder doesn't have to be fancy, but it should be sturdy and grind smoothly. While you're at it, a second pepper grinder or a spice mill is nice to have for grinding whole spices.

Plastic refrigerator-freezer containers. I recommend cooking large batches of foods that freeze well so you will always have a low-fat meal on hand when you're in a hurry or aren't in the mood to cook. It's easy if you have a large assortment of freezer containers with tight-fitting lids. Keep a roll of masking tape or freezer tape and a marking pencil handy so you can label each dish with the contents and date.

Sushi rolling mat. You'll only need this if you plan to make sushi (page 183). I haven't found any other use for mine. It's just a lot of thin bamboo sticks tied together into a mat about one foot square. You can buy one in an Asian grocery store.

Toaster and toaster oven. I use these constantly to toast pita bread and French bread. Breads made without fat have a very short shelf-life. Keep pita bread in the refrigerator or freezer. French bread is best the same day it's bought, but if you have a stale piece, you can bring it back to life by sprinkling it with a few drops of water and warming it in a toaster oven.

Basic Quinoa

> 1 cup quinoa
> 2 cups bouillon (see page 187)

Bring the bouillon to a boil, stir in the quinoa and return to boiling. Reduce the heat, cover and simmer 10 to 15 minutes, or until the liquid is absorbed and the quinoa is transparent and tender.

Quinoa can also be toasted before cooking. Follow the instructions for millet, above.

About 2 cups

Spanish Rice

Pair Spanish rice with beans, or serve it with broiled fish. Add a green salad or a steamed green vegetable and you have a whole meal.

> 1 cup brown rice
> 1 onion, chopped
> 1 green pepper, chopped
> 1 sweet red pepper, chopped
> 2 stalks celery, chopped
> 3 cups bouillon (see page 187)
> 1 can (28 ounces) plum tomatoes, chopped
> 1 tablespoon fresh oregano or 1 teaspoon dried
> ½ teaspoon saffron or ½ teaspoon turmeric
> 1 bay leaf
> Pinch cayenne or to taste
> 8 ounces mushrooms, sliced
> 2 cups frozen peas
> 1 can artichoke hearts, drained and cut in pieces
> ½ cup Italian parsley, chopped
> Juice of 1 lemon
> Freshly ground black pepper

Combine the rice, onion, peppers, celery, bouillon, tomatoes and seasonings; bring to a boil and simmer, covered, 30 minutes. Add the mushrooms and continue to simmer 10 minutes. Stir in the peas and artichoke hearts; simmer 5 minutes more, or until the rice is tender and has absorbed most of the liquid. Stir in the parsley and lemon juice and serve with ground black pepper to taste.

4 to 6 servings

Rosy Rice

This easy rice dish is great with black beans and a green salad.

> 1 large onion, chopped
> 3 cloves garlic, minced
> 1 cup brown rice
> 2½ cups bouillon (see page 187)
> 1 can (28 ounces) plum tomatoes, chopped
> 1 teaspoon ground cumin
> 1 bay leaf
> 1 teaspoon oregano

Combine all the ingredients; bring to a boil and simmer 45 minutes, covered, or until the rice is tender and most of the liquid is absorbed.

4 servings

Arroz Verde

If you want a special rice dish to accompany one of my vegetable chilis, try this. It's also good with steamed shrimp.

> 1 cup brown rice
> 2½ cups bouillon (see page 187)
> ½ teaspoon dry mustard
> 1 green pepper, chopped
> 2 cans (4 ounces each) green chiles, drained and chopped
> ¼ cup cilantro leaves, chopped
> Freshly ground black pepper

Combine the rice, bouillon, mustard and green pepper and bring to a boil. Reduce the heat and simmer, covered, until the rice is tender, about 45 minutes. Stir in the green chiles and cilantro and serve with ground black pepper to taste.

4 servings

Red Pepper Pilaf

Roasting or broiling sweet red peppers brings out the flavor and adds a smokey note. Combine them with rice and you get a pilaf that's both colorful and tasty.

> 3 cups bouillon (see page 187)
> 1 cup brown rice
> 1 large sweet red pepper
> 1 onion, chopped
> Freshly ground black pepper

Set aside ½ cup of the bouillon. Bring the remaining 2½ cups to a boil and stir in the brown rice; cover, reduce the heat and cook 40 to 45 minutes, or until tender but not mushy. Meanwhile, cook the onion in the reserved ½ cup of bouillon until softened, about 10 minutes. Roast the pepper over a gas flame or under a broiler until the skin is charred. Place it in a paper bag to cool. Remove the seeds, stem and most of the skin and chop the pepper into small dice. When the rice is cooked, stir in the red pepper and onion. Season to taste with ground black pepper.

4 servings

Orange Rice

I like to use fruit in unexpected ways, not just for dessert. Here, sweet chunks of orange provide just the right contrast for spicy bean or seafood dishes.

> 1½ cups orange juice
> 1 cup water
> ½ teaspoon salt
> ½ cup chopped green onions
> ½ cup chopped celery
> 1 cup brown rice
> 2 oranges, peeled and cubed

Bring the juice, water, salt, onion and celery to a boil and simmer 5 minutes. Add the rice; cover and simmer 40 minutes, or until the rice is tender and the liquid is absorbed. Stir in the orange chunks.

4 servings

Cumin Seed Rice

Whole cumin seeds give this rice dish distinction. It's perfect to accompany beans or vegetable chilis.

> 1 onion, chopped
> 1 green pepper, chopped
> 2 stalks celery, chopped
> 2 cloves garlic, minced
> 1 dried red pepper, crumbled
> 1 can (28 ounces) plum tomatoes
> 3½ cups bouillon (see page 187)
> 1½ cups brown rice
> 1 tablespoon whole cumin seed

Bring all the ingredients except the rice and cumin seed to a boil and simmer 5 minutes. Stir, breaking up the tomatoes. Add the rice and cumin seed. Simmer, covered, 40 minutes, or until the rice is tender.

6 to 8 servings

Ginger Rice

Brown rice takes on an oriental flair with gingerroot, garlic and spinach. Try it with steamed fish fillets.

> 1 cup brown rice
> 2½ cups bouillon (see page 187)
> 2 cloves garlic, minced
> 2 tablespoons grated gingerroot
> 1 pound spinach, torn into pieces or 10 ounces frozen spinach
> Freshly ground black pepper

Bring the rice, bouillon, garlic and gingerroot to a boil and simmer, covered, 40 minutes, or until the rice is tender but not mushy. Meanwhile, steam the spinach until it is wilted. If using frozen spinach, cook it according to the package directions. Combine the spinach with the cooked rice and serve with ground black pepper to taste.

4 to 6 servings

Wild Rice with Shiitake Mushrooms

The mild anise flavor of fennel blends with the woodsy mushrooms for an outstanding side dish. Any leftovers make an equally exceptional salad.

1 onion, chopped
2 cloves garlic, minced
1 fennel bulb, chopped
4 cups bouillon (see page 187)
1 cup wild rice
Pinch cayenne or to taste
½ cup shiitake or other mushrooms, sliced
½ cup Italian parsley, chopped
Freshly ground black pepper

Bring the onion, garlic, fennel and bouillon to a boil. Stir in the wild rice and cayenne; cover, reduce the heat and simmer 20 minutes. Add the mushrooms; cover and continue cooking 30 to 40 minutes, or until the rice is tender. Stir in the parsley and season with ground black pepper to taste.

6 to 8 servings

Confetti Rice

You can stretch wild rice by combining it with brown rice and dressing it up with petite peas and mushrooms. This recipe makes enough for a holiday meal. Leftovers are delicious reheated or made into a salad. For a special variation (warm or cold), stir in a 4-ounce can of tiny cocktail shrimp.

5½ cups bouillon, divided (see page 187)
1 cup wild rice
1 cup brown rice
1 teaspoon ground cumin
8 ounces mushrooms, sliced
1 cup frozen petite peas

Bring 3 cups of the bouillon to a boil; add the wild rice, cover and simmer 1 hour. Fifteen minutes after you start the wild rice, bring the remaining 2½ cups of bouillon to a boil in another pot, add the brown rice and cumin. Cover and simmer 35 to 40 minutes, or until tender. Put the frozen peas in a strainer and run warm water over them to thaw. About 5 minutes before the wild rice is done, add the sliced mushrooms to it. Drain the wild rice if necessary; combine the two rices in a serving bowl and stir in the peas.

8 to 10 servings

Barley and Wild Mushrooms

Barley cooked this way reminds me of risotto, the Italian specialty made with short-grain refined rice (and lots of fat).

> ½ cup pearl barley
> 3½ cups bouillon (see page 187)
> 1 onion, chopped
> 1 clove garlic, minced
> ½ pound shiitake mushrooms or other wild mushrooms
> ½ cup white wine (optional)
> ¼ cup fresh basil leaves or Italian parsley, chopped

Bring 3 cups of the bouillon to a boil and stir in the barley. Cover, reduce the heat and simmer 30 to 40 minutes, or until the barley is tender; drain if necessary. Meanwhile, cook the onion and garlic in the remaining ½ cup bouillon until softened, about 10 minutes. Add the mushrooms and wine, if desired, and simmer 5 minutes. Stir the vegetables into the barley and sprinkle with basil or parsley.

4 servings

Bulgur with Greens

You can combine bulgur with any greens that appeal to you. Once you've tried the basic recipe, try varying it with spices.

> 1 onion, chopped
> 2 cloves garlic, minced
> 1 dried red pepper, crumbled
> 2 cups bouillon (see page 187)
> 1 cup bulgur
> 4 cups Swiss chard, escarole or spinach, chopped
> Freshly ground black pepper

Bring the onion, garlic, pepper and bouillon to a boil and simmer 5 minutes. Return to a boil; stir in the bulgur and escarole. Simmer, covered, 20 to 25 minutes. Remove from the heat and let stand 10 minutes. Fluff with a fork and serve with ground black pepper to taste.

4 to 6 servings

Fennel, Bulgur and Peas

This time bulgur that is teamed with fennel, bits of red pepper and tiny bright green peas.

> *1 fennel bulb*
> *1 sweet red pepper, chopped*
> *1 cup sliced green onions*
> *2 cloves garlic, minced*
> *2 cups bouillon (see page 187)*
> *1 cup bulgur*
> *2 cups frozen baby peas, defrosted*
> *Freshly ground black pepper*

Chop the fennel bulb and stalks into ½-inch pieces; reserve the leaves. Bring the chopped fennel, red pepper, onion, garlic and bouillon to a boil; reduce the heat and simmer 5 minutes. Stir in the bulgur and simmer, covered, 20 to 25 minutes, or until tender. Snip the reserved fennel leaves into tiny pieces and stir them in along with the peas. Remove from the heat and let stand 10 minutes. Fluff with a fork and serve with ground black pepper to taste.

4 to 6 servings

Bulgur Dumplings

Any soup will be improved with the addition of these light, egg-free dumplings.

> *1½ cups hot water*
> *1 cup bulgur*
> *1 cup whole-wheat flour*
> *½ teaspoon salt*
> *Simmering broth or soup*

Place the bulgur in a bowl; pour hot water over it and let stand at least 10 minutes. Squeeze out the excess liquid. Add the flour and salt and let stand at least 5 minutes. Scoop out marble-size pieces with a teaspoon and drop into simmering bouillon or the soup of your choice. Cover and simmer 20 minutes.

Enough dumplings for 6 to 8 servings of soup

Oatmeal Stew

Don't confine oatmeal to the breakfast table. Try cooking and seasoning it as you do other whole grains, and I think you'll be pleasantly surprised. It's good for thickening soups; here, it makes a tasty side dish that's especially nice with fish.

> 1 onion, chopped
> 2 cloves garlic, minced
> 1 dried red pepper, crumbled
> 4 cups bouillon (see page 187)
> 1 potato, diced
> 1 fennel bulb, chopped
> 1 cup rolled oats (not quick-cooking)
> 1 pound spinach, chopped
> 1/2 teaspoon nutmeg
> 1/4 teaspoon allspice
> Freshly ground black pepper

Cook the onion, garlic and red pepper in bouillon until softened, about 10 minutes. Add the potato and fennel and simmer 15 minutes. Stir in the oatmeal, spinach and seasonings and cook 10 minutes. Puree half the stew in a blender; stir it back into the pot and reheat. Serve with ground black pepper to taste.

4 to 6 servings

Orzo Pepper Pilaf

A baked orzo pilaf makes a nice occasional change from rice. Flecks of red and yellow pepper brighten up your plate.

> 2 tablespoons lemon juice
> 1 small red onion, chopped
> 2 cloves garlic, minced
> 1 small sweet red pepper, chopped
> 1 small yellow bell pepper, chopped
> ¼ cup Italian parsley, chopped
> 1 tablespoon fresh oregano or ½ teaspoon dried
> 2 cups cooked orzo (rice-shaped pasta)

Preheat the oven to 350°F. Cook the onion, garlic and peppers in the lemon juice until softened, about 5 minutes. Combine with the remaining ingredients in a baking dish; cover and bake 30 minutes.

4 to 6 servings

Dilly Potatoes

Don't peel the potatoes, just scrub them. If you can get tiny new potatoes, by all means use them in this recipe.

> 4 red potatoes
> ½ cup bouillon
> ½ cup fresh dillweed, chopped
> 3 garlic cloves, halved
> Freshly ground black pepper

Cut the potatoes into bite-size chunks. Bring the bouillon to a boil; add the potatoes, dillweed and garlic. Reduce the heat; cover and steam 15 minutes, or until the potatoes are just tender. Remove the garlic, if desired, and serve with ground black pepper to taste.

4 servings

New Potato Curry

This curry is on the borderline between a main dish and a side dish. If you add some beans, there won't be any question. I like to serve it with two or three other curried dishes, chutney and raita (see pages 284–286) for a glorious Indian-inspired buffet.

>2 pounds new potatoes or small red potatoes
>½ cup bouillon (see page 187)
>1 onion, chopped
>1 jalapeño pepper, seeded and chopped
>2 teaspoons curry powder
>1 teaspoon grated gingerroot
>½ teaspoon whole cumin seed
>½ teaspoon fennel seed
>¼ cup cilantro, chopped
>3 ripe tomatoes, chopped, or 2 cups canned
>1 cup frozen baby peas, thawed (optional)

Boil the potatoes until just tender; halve or quarter into bite-size pieces. While the potatoes cook, heat the bouillon and cook the onion, pepper and spices until softened, about 10 minutes. Stir in the tomatoes and half of the cilantro and cook 5 minutes. Add the potatoes and peas and cook a few minutes to heat through. Sprinkle with the remaining cilantro.

6 to 8 servings

Potatoes with Green Chile Salsa

If you like this combination, try topping a baked potato with salsa.

>6 red potatoes
>1 green pepper, chopped
>4 green onions, chopped
>1 cup green chile salsa (see page 312)

Boil the potatoes until just tender, about 20 minutes. Cool, dice and combine with the green pepper and green onions. Stir in the salsa and chill 30 minutes.

4 to 6 servings

Yam-Apple Bake

I love something sweet to eat right along with spicy foods, but you could just as easily serve my Yam-Apple Bake for dessert.

> *4 apples, peeled, cored and sliced thin*
> *4 yams or sweet potatoes, peeled and sliced thin*
> *¼ cup apple cider*
> *1 tablespoon lemon juice*
> *1 teaspoon cinnamon*
> *¼ cup brown sugar*

Preheat the oven to 350°F. Combine all of the ingredients except the brown sugar in a casserole and bake, covered 1 hour. Remove the cover, sprinkle with the brown sugar and bake 15 more minutes.

4 to 6 servings

Vegetable Side Dishes

A side dish of crisp-tender cooked vegetables adds tremendous appeal to a meal of beans and grains or seafood. Just about any vegetable imaginable can be cooked by steaming in about ½ cup of liquid (water, bouillon, wine or juice) until it is just tender. The cardinal rule for vegetables is . . . don't overcook. They quickly become mushy and uninteresting and lose their bright colors.

Single vegetables are good, but combinations are better. Experiment with two, three or more vegetables that have complementary colors and textures. They'll be even more interesting if you add spices or fresh herbs.

This section contains some of my favorite vegetable side dishes to get you started. Don't hesitate to change the recipes, varying the vegetables and seasonings to suit your taste and to take advantage of whatever looks good in the produce department.

Mock Stir-Fry Veggies

Chinese stir-fried vegetables are delicious, but you don't need the added oil. You can get the same bright, crispy vegetables by cooking them quickly in a little bouillon.

> *½ cup bouillon or clam juice*
> *2 carrots, sliced thin*
> *1 onion, sliced*
> *1 clove garlic, minced*
> *1 teaspoon grated gingerroot*
> *1 can (8 ounces) sliced water chestnuts, drained*
> *½ pound snow peas (fresh or frozen)*
> *1 pound fresh spinach, washed*
> *1 tablespoon soy sauce*
> *1 teaspoon cornstarch*

In a large covered saucepan, heat the bouillon to boiling and cook the carrots, onion, garlic and gingerroot until the vegetables are softened, about 10 minutes. Add the water chestnuts and snow peas. Mix the soy sauce and cornstarch; stir it into the vegetables and cook 2 minutes. Add the spinach; cover and cook until it is just wilted, about 2 minutes.

4 to 6 servings

Roasted Vegetable Medley

You have your choice of cooking methods here. I like to roast the vegetables in the oven, but you can cook them outdoors on a grill just as easily. Or you can just steam them in a covered pan on the stovetop.

> *2 zucchini, halved lengthwise and cut into ½-inch slices*
> *1 sweet red pepper, chopped*
> *1 green pepper, chopped*
> *½ pound mushrooms, halved*
> *1 cup pearl onions (frozen ones are convenient) or 1 onion, chopped*
> *2 stalks celery, cut in ½-inch slices*
> *2 tablespoons Worcestershire sauce*
> *1 teaspoon snipped fresh tarragon*
> *1 teaspoon grated lemon peel*

Preheat the oven to 400° F. Place the vegetables on a large sheet of aluminum foil and sprinkle with Worcestershire sauce and seasonings.

Fold the foil around the vegetables, seal the edges and roast them 15 minutes. Be careful when you open the foil — steam can burn.

4 servings

Root Roast

The vegetables in this foil-roasted packet take longer to cook than the preceding combination, but the principle is the same. You could cook them on an outdoor grill or steam them in a pot.

> *2 onions, peeled and cut into chunks*
> *4 carrots, quartered lengthwise and cut into 2-inch pieces*
> *8 small red potatoes, quartered*
> *2 tablespoons minced fresh marjoram or 1 teaspoon dried*
> *1 tablespoon fresh rosemary leaves or ½ teaspoon dried*
> *4 cloves garlic, minced*
> *Freshly ground black pepper to taste*

Preheat the oven to 425° F. Arrange the vegetables on a large sheet of heavy foil and sprinkle them with the seasonings and minced garlic. Seal the foil and bake 45 minutes. Remove the packet from the oven, shake it gently and open it up. Return it to the oven and bake an additional 10 minutes. Serve with additional ground black pepper to taste.

4 servings

Ratatouille

Eggplant, tomatoes, peppers and onions are the essential ingredients of ratatouille. Beyond that, you can add and subtract vegetables and herbs to your heart's content. Ratatouille is equally good warm, at room temperature or chilled. It tastes even better the second day and freezes well, so make lots.

> *1 onion, chopped*
> *1 green pepper, chopped*
> *4 stalks celery, chopped*
> *4 cloves garlic, minced*
> *½ cup bouillon (see page 187)*

2 cups green beans, cut in 1-inch pieces
1 large eggplant, cubed
1 can (28 ounces) plum tomatoes, chopped
¼ cup fresh basil leaves, chopped
1 bay leaf
2 tablespoons lemon juice
2 tablespoons capers
Freshly ground black pepper

Cook the onion, peppers, celery and garlic in the bouillon to soften, about 5 minutes. Add the beans, eggplant, tomatoes, basil and bay leaf; cover and simmer 20 minutes or until the vegetables are tender and the flavors are blended, stirring occasionally and adding more liquid if necessary. Stir in the lemon juice and capers and serve with ground black pepper to taste.

8 to 10 servings

Ginger-Steamed Vegetables

If you keep a piece of gingerroot in your refrigerator, you'll always be ready to deliver a gourmet vegetable dish. This recipe works with just about any combination of crisp-textured vegetables.

1 small head cauliflower, broken into florets
2 carrots, cut in ½-inch pieces
2 small zucchini, sliced
2 teaspoons grated fresh gingerroot
½ cup bouillon (see page 187)

Bring the bouillon to a boil; add the vegetables and ginger. Reduce the heat; cover and steam 10 to 15 minutes, or until the carrots and cauliflower are crisp-tender.

4 servings

Lemon Green Beans

Before you buy fresh beans for this recipe, snap the end off 1 to make sure they are young and tender. Otherwise, frozen ones work just fine.

½ cup bouillon (see page 187)
1 pound green beans in 1-inch pieces (fresh or frozen)
1 can (8 ounces) sliced water chestnuts, rinsed
½ cup pearl onions (frozen ones are easy to use)
2 tablespoons lemon juice
1 teaspoon grated lemon peel
Freshly ground black pepper to taste

Place all the ingredients in a pot. Bring to a boil, reduce the heat, and simmer 6 to 8 minutes, or until the beans are crisp-tender. Serve with additional ground pepper to taste.

4 to 6 servings

Mint-Glazed Carrots

Sometimes fresh carrots aren't as sweet as I'd like them to be; the brown sugar helps. Save a few whole mint leaves for a pretty garnish.

½ cup bouillon (see page 187)
4 to 6 carrots, sliced
2 teaspoons cornstarch
¼ cup brown sugar
¼ cup fresh mint leaves, chopped

Bring the bouillon to a boil; add the carrots and simmer 8 to 10 minutes, or until tender. Remove the carrots with a slotted spoon. Mix the cornstarch and brown sugar in a bowl; gradually stir in the cooking liquid. Return the mixture to the pot and bring to a boil, stirring constantly until thickened. Stir in the carrots and chopped mint.

4 servings

Mexican-Style Corn

What can you do with corn on the cob when you give up butter? Here's my solution.

> 4 ears corn on the cob
> ½ cup nonfat Italian dressing
> 1 tablespoon chili powder

Cook the corn in boiling water to cover until tender, about 5 minutes. Combine the dressing and chili powder and brush on the corn.

4 servings

Bettejane's Acorn Squash with Applesauce

Why waste time baking when squash cooks so quickly in a microwave?

> 2 acorn squash
> 2 cups applesauce
> ¼ cup raisins
> ¼ teaspoon nutmeg

Cook the squash at the high setting in a microwave oven 2 minutes. Cut them in half and scoop out the seeds. Combine the remaining ingredients and spoon into the squash halves; cook in the microwave 4 to 5 minutes, or until the squash is tender.

4 servings

Sweet and Sour Cabbage

This refreshing side dish is served in some Chinese restaurants. It's not quite a salad and not quite a cooked vegetable.

> 1 small head cabbage
> ½ cup water
> ½ cup cider vinegar
> 6 tablespoons sugar
> Juice of 1 lemon
> ½ teaspoon salt

Slice the cabbage into ¼-inch strips. Bring the water to a boil and add the cabbage; cover and steam 5 minutes, or until the cabbage is crisp-tender. Rinse with cold water and drain. Combine the remaining ingredients and toss with the cabbage. Chill at least 20 minutes.

4 to 6 servings

Swiss Chard with Leeks

Sometimes you can find "rhubarb" Swiss chard, which has bright red ribs. It tastes just like regular chard (not at all like rhubarb), and the color is sensational.

> *4 leeks, sliced*
> *3 stalks celery, chopped*
> *1 clove garlic, minced*
> *¼ cup bouillon (see page 187)*
> *1 pound Swiss chard, chopped*
> *Freshly ground black pepper*

Cook the leeks, celery and garlic in the bouillon 10 minutes to soften. Add the Swiss chard; cover and steam 5 minutes or until the chard is wilted. Season with freshly ground black pepper to taste.

4 to 6 servings

Spinach Adobo

Spinach was never my favorite vegetable, but I don't complain when it's steamed with garlic and soy sauce.

> *3 cloves garlic, minced*
> *3 tablespoons soy sauce*
> *1 tablespoon rice wine vinegar*
> *1 pound spinach, rinsed and chopped*
> *Freshly ground black pepper*

Cook the garlic, soy sauce and vinegar in a saucepan over low heat 5 minutes. Stir in the spinach; cover and steam 3 to 4 minutes, or just until wilted. Serve with ground black pepper to taste.

4 servings

Vegetables with Cellophane Noodles

Cellophane noodles cook quickly and add an interesting texture to this vegetable dish.

> 3 ounces cellophane noodles
> 2 onions, chopped
> 2 small zucchini, diced
> 1 green pepper, chopped
> 1 can (16 ounces) plum tomatoes, chopped
> 1 tablespoon lemon juice
> Soy sauce

Soak the noodles in cold water to cover 10 minutes. Combine the vegetables, bring to a boil, lower the heat and cook 10 minutes, or until the onion and pepper are softened. Stir in the noodles and cook 2 to 3 minutes. Season with lemon juice and soy sauce to taste.

4 servings

Relishes and Condiments

When you take away fat, you need to find lots of other ways to make food taste good. Relishes and condiments add sweet tastes to contrast with spicy food, tart tastes to complement mellow foods, or hot and spicy tastes to perk up bland dishes. Contrast is the key!

Fortunately, most relishes, pickles and condiments in your supermarket are made without fat. You can use all the mustard, ketchup and pickles you want. Explore the ethnic food sections for other interesting condiments. Just check the labels to make sure they are made without oil.

You can expand the variety of condiments on your table by making some of your own. For example, chutneys can be made from a variety of fruits, and they are very easy to cook. Try these recipes and then invent some of your own.

Peach Chutney

Chutney is exceptionally easy to make if you use canned fruit. Don't be put off by the long list of ingredients in these three chutney recipes; you just go through your spice shelf and assemble them in minutes.

4 cups sliced fresh, frozen or canned peaches
1 cup raisins
¼ cup lemon juice
1½ cups sugar
¼ cup vinegar
1 teaspoon ground cumin
Pinch cayenne or to taste
½ teaspoon dried thyme
1 teaspoon cinnamon
10 black peppercorns
1 teaspoon fennel seed
1 teaspoon coriander seed
½ teaspoon mustard seed

Stir the peaches, raisins and lemon juice together in a bowl. Combine the remaining ingredients in a large saucepan and boil gently 12 to 15 minutes, or until thick. (If using canned peaches, add some of the syrup instead of the sugar.) Add the fruit and simmer about 1 to 3 minutes. Let the flavors blend at least an hour and preferably overnight. Keeps well, refrigerated in sealed containers.

About 4 cups

Apple-Pear Chutney

4 Granny Smith or other tart apples, cored and chopped
2 pears, cored and chopped
½ cup golden raisins
2 cloves garlic, minced
2 tablespoons grated gingerroot
1 teaspoon cinnamon
1 teaspoon ground cardamom
1 teaspoon ground allspice
Pinch cayenne or to taste
½ cup cider vinegar
¼ cup lemon juice

Combine the ingredients and simmer, covered, for 20 minutes, or until the apples are tender but not mushy. Refrigerate in tightly covered containers.

About 3 cups

Pineapple Chutney

>   1 cup sugar
>   ¼ cup vinegar
>   1 teaspoon cinnamon
>   Pinch cayenne or to taste
>   1 teaspoon fennel seed
>   1 pineapple, peeled, cored and cut into ½-inch chunks, or 3 cups canned, drained
>   ½ cup golden raisins

Combine the sugar, vinegar, cinnamon, cayenne and fennel seed in a large saucepan and boil gently 12 to 15 minutes, or until thick. Add the pineapple and raisins; simmer 5 to 10 minutes. Let the flavors blend at least an hour and preferably overnight. Keeps well, refrigerated in sealed containers.

About 3 cups

Spiced Apple Rings

You can tint these with red food coloring, if you like, to make a garnish that's pretty as well as tasty.

>   4 apples, cored and sliced
>   ½ cup brown sugar
>   1 teaspoon cinnamon
>   ¼ teaspoon ground cloves
>   ¼ teaspoon ground ginger

Combine all the ingredients in a saucepan; heat and stir gently until the apples are soft, about 15 minutes.

About 3 cups

Cucumber Raita

Raitas are Indian in origin. They all start with yogurt and add other ingredients such as cucumbers, chiles or potatoes. They're refreshing served with spicy curries or chilis, and make good salad dressings. Here are two combinations; you can invent others.

> 1 cup plain nonfat yogurt
> 2 cucumbers, peeled and diced
> 4 cloves garlic, minced
> 1 cup cilantro, chopped
> Pinch cayenne or to taste

Combine all the ingredients.

About 2 cups

Green Chile Raita

> 1 cup plain nonfat yogurt
> 5 mild green chiles, roasted, seeded and chopped (see page 138), or use canned chiles
> 2 cucumbers, peeled and diced
> ½ cup cilantro, chopped
> 6 scallions, sliced
> 2 cloves garlic, minced
> 2 tablespoons lime juice or vinegar

Combine all the ingredients.

About 2 cups

Spicy Onion Relish

Try my spicy onion relish with vegetable chilies, curries or broiled fish. A little goes a long way.

> 1 onion, chopped
> 2 tablespoons lime or lemon juice
> ½ teaspoon cayenne or to taste
> Salt to taste

Combine all the ingredients and refrigerate at least 30 minutes. Keeps well.

About 1 cup

Caponata

This eggplant relish is wonderful with fish. It also makes a good appetizer, served with pita toasts.

> 1 medium eggplant
> 1 green pepper, chopped
> 1 medium onion, chopped
> 4 cloves garlic, minced
> 8 ounces mushrooms, sliced
> 1 can (6 ounces) tomato paste
> 1/2 teaspoon red pepper flakes
> 1/2 teaspoon oregano
> 1/2 teaspoon salt
> 1/4 cup wine vinegar
> 1/4 cup water

Roast the eggplant over a gas flame or under a broiler until the skin is charred and the flesh is soft, about 10 minutes. Rub off most of the skin; chop the flesh and combine it with the remaining ingredients. Simmer gently 15 to 20 minutes. Let stand at least an hour to let the flavors blend or refrigerate overnight. Serve at room temperature or chilled.

About 3 cups

Giardiniera

Mixed pickled vegetables can be made up in large batches because they keep well in the refrigerator. You can use any combination of vegetables you like.

> 2 carrots, sliced diagonally
> 2 stalks celery, sliced diagonally
> 2 cups cauliflower florets
> 1 sweet red pepper, sliced
> 4 green onions, sliced (white part only)
> 2 cloves garlic, minced
> 1 cup wine vinegar
> 1/2 cup water
> 1 teaspoon salt
> 1/4 teaspoon red pepper flakes or to taste
> 10 peppercorns
> Sprig of dillweed (optional)

Mix all the ingredients and refrigerate, covered, for 2 days before serving.

About 4 cups

Fruits and Dessert Treats

Fruit is by far the best dessert for a low-fat diet. With so many kinds to choose from, you'll never get bored. Best of all, you don't have to limit yourself. You can have this dessert with breakfast, lunch, and dinner and anytime in between.

You may think that fruit is fine for your own meals but too boring for guests. It doesn't have to be! With so many exotic fruits available year-round in our supermarkets, you can always create a glamorous compote with varicolored fruits in a glass bowl. Use your imagination to come up with new combinations, concentrating on the basic principles of contrast — color, texture and flavor. In the cold months, cooked or spiced fruits are particularly appealing.

If you make angel food cake, fruit breads and other nonfat baked desserts, remember that they are made with sugar and refined flour that has very little fiber. You need to count each portion as 1 of your 5 daily servings of low-fat/low-fiber foods.

Be especially careful if you buy "nonfat" bakery products. Check the portion size and the calories. Manufacturers have figured out how to make delicious pastries with artificial fats, but these delights have very little fiber and lots of calories — and they taste so good, you'll want to eat the whole thing. Remember, your body converts all extra calories to fat. These "nonfat" treats must be counted in your daily tally of 5 servings of low-fiber foods. A "serving" may be no bigger than your finger!

Poached Pears

Cranberry juice turns the pears a lovely bright pink.

> 4 ripe pears, halved and cored
> 1/2 cup golden raisins
> 2 cups cranberry juice
> 1/2 teaspoon cinnamon
> 6 whole cloves
> Grated rind of 1 orange

Combine all the ingredients in a saucepan and bring to a boil. Simmer, covered, for 15 minutes, or until the pears are just tender.

4 servings

Spiced Melon

Coriander and nutmeg bring out the best in melon. When picking out melons, remember that if it doesn't smell sweet, it probably won't have much flavor. This technique doesn't apply to watermelons — they're always a gamble.

> 8 cups melon balls (mix your favorite kinds)
> 2 tablespoons lime juice
> 2 tablespoons honey
> ¼ teaspoon ground coriander
> ¼ teaspoon ground nutmeg
> Fresh mint leaves

Combine all the ingredients and chill at least 30 minutes.

4 servings

Baked Apples

These apples smell so good while they're cooking, you'll have a hard time staying out of the kitchen.

> 1 cup brown sugar
> Juice of ½ lemon
> ¼ cup raisins
> 1 teaspoon cinnamon
> 4 large, firm apples, cored

Preheat the oven to 350° F. Mix the sugar, lemon juice, raisins and cinnamon. Arrange the apples in a baking dish lined with foil and fill the cores with the raisin mixture. Sprinkle any remaining raisin mixture around the apples and bake 1 hour. Serve warm or cold.

4 servings

Pineapple Fruit Boats

Fruit-filled pineapples work with any combination of your favorite fruit. They're prettiest if you have brightly contrasting colors. For a special treat, marinate the fruit in ¼ cup of liqueur or fruit syrup.

> 1 fresh pineapple
> 1 cup raspberries
> 1 cup green grapes, halved
> 1 cup blueberries
> ¼ cup fruit-flavored liqueur or fruit syrup (optional)

Slice the pineapple in half lengthwise. Remove the fruit, leaving the shell and leaves intact. Cut away the core; dice the pineapple and mix it with the other fruits. Stir in the liqueur or syrup, if desired, and spoon into the pineapple shells.

2 to 4 servings

Gingered Fruit Compote

Candied ginger turns just about any mixture of fruits into party fare. You'll find it in the Asian or gourmet section of the supermarket or in Asian groceries.

> 4 slices candied ginger
> 1 small pineapple, peeled, cored and cut in bite-size pieces
> 2 bananas, peeled and sliced
> 1 cup seedless grapes, halved
> 2 large or 4 small tangerines, peeled and sectioned

Cut the candied ginger into ¼-inch slivers. Combine with all the fruits in a pretty glass bowl. Chill until ready to serve.

4 servings

Glazed Bananas

You can count on finding fresh bananas year-round. I like this best on a cold, wintery day.

> 6 bananas
> ½ cup brown sugar
> ½ teaspoon cinnamon

Preheat the broiler. Cover a cookie sheet with foil. Peel the bananas, slice them in half lengthwise, then cut each half in three pieces cross-ways. Arrange the banana pieces close together in a single layer on the cookie sheet. Mix the brown sugar and cinnamon together and sprinkle over the bananas. Broil the bananas about 3 to 4 minutes, until the sugar bubbles and the bananas are nicely glazed.

4 servings

Ginger-Pear Frappe

I encourage you to experiment with frozen and partially frozen fruit — as dessert ingredients or snacks.

> 1 can (29 ounces) pear halves
> 4 slices candied ginger
> ½ cup orange juice

Drain the pears and freeze them until firm. Cut the candied ginger into small dice. Thaw the pear halves for 10 to 15 minutes and cut into pieces. Place in a blender or food processor with 1 teaspoon of the ginger and the orange juice; blend until smooth. Serve immediately, garnished with the remaining candied ginger.

4 to 6 servings

Easy Banana-Strawberry Sorbet

Here's another good trick with frozen fruits — a sorbet worthy of the finest restaurant.

> 4 bananas
> 1 cup sliced strawberries, fresh or frozen
> ½ cup tropical fruit punch or guava drink
> Additional strawberries for garnish

Peel the bananas, place in a plastic bag and freeze until firm. When ready to serve, slice the bananas into chunks. Place the bananas, 1 cup of strawberries and the fruit punch in a blender or food processor and puree until smooth. Garnish with the remaining strawberries.

4 servings

Fruit Kabobs

Fruit kabobs can be broiled, or you can just thread a variety of fresh fruit chunks on skewers and serve as they are.

> 2 slightly green bananas, cut in 1-inch pieces
> 1 cup fresh or canned pineapple chunks
> 4 star fruit, cut in ¼-inch slices
> 1 papaya, peeled and cut into 1-inch cubes
> 2 tablespoons lime juice
> 2 tablespoons lemon juice
> ¼ cup honey

Arrange the chunks of fruit on skewers. Combine the juices with the h1y and brush on the kabobs. Broil for about 3 minutes; turn and baste, and broil 2 more minutes.

4 servings

Angel Food Cake with Ginger-Apricot Sauce

Angel food cakes are almost always fat free, so if you're on a tight schedule and need a fancy dessert, you can buy one in the bakery section and dress it up with a spicy fruit sauce.

1 can (16 ounces) apricot halves in light syrup
1 teaspoon grated fresh gingerroot
2 teaspoons cornstarch
1 angel food cake, purchased or made from a mix

Puree the apricots and ½ cup of their juice in a blender. In a small bowl, mix the cornstarch, ginger and 2 tablespoons of the apricot juice until smooth. Combine the apricot puree and cornstarch mixture in a saucepan; bring to a boil and cook 1 minute, or until thickened, stirring constantly. Serve warm (or room temperature) over angel food cake slices.

8 servings

Pineapple Fruit Cake

I invented my pineapple cake for a holiday party, but it's simple enough to make anytime. Try it with other canned or dry fruits, too.

1½ cups flour
1 cup quick-cooking oatmeal
1 teaspoon baking powder
1 teaspoon baking soda
1 teaspoon cinnamon
½ teaspoon nutmeg
½ cup light brown sugar, divided
1 can (20 ounces) pineapple tidbits
1 cup golden raisins
1 cup apple butter

Preheat the oven to 350°F. Mix the flour, oatmeal, baking powder, baking soda, cinnamon, nutmeg, and ¼ cup of the brown sugar together in a large bowl.

Prepare the baking pan: Pat the remaining ¼ cup of brown sugar evenly over the bottom of a 5-by-9-inch nonstick loaf pan. Drain the pineapple and arrange several of the pieces on the brown sugar in the bottom of the pan.

Stir the remaining pineapple tidbits, the raisins and apple butter into the dry ingredients in the mixing bowl. Blend well and pour into the baking pan. Bake 1 hour. Remove from the oven, invert on a serving plate and allow to cool. After about 10 minutes, you should be able to lift the baking pan off the cake. The cake can be cut into thin slices after it cools.

8 servings

Banana Bread

My fat- and egg-free banana bread may be heavier than most, but it's delicious just the same.

> 6 *very ripe bananas*
> 1 *cup sugar*
> 2 *cups flour*
> 1 *teaspoon baking powder*
> ½ *teaspoon baking soda*
> 1 *teaspoon vanilla*
> 1 *cup golden raisins*

Preheat the oven to 350°F. Mash the bananas and sugar together. In a separate bowl, mix the flour, baking powder and baking soda. Stir in the banana mixture and the vanilla; when thoroughly blended, add the raisins. Pour into a nonstick loaf pan and bake 1 hour. Cool slightly and remove from the pan; allow to cool completely before slicing.

8 servings

Fruity Oatmeal Bars

Apple butter is the secret ingredient in these tasty treats. You can eat them for dessert, as a snack or even for breakfast on-the-run. My favorites are made with dates and apricots, but you can use any dried fruit or combination of fruits — raisins, apples, figs, peaches or some of the more exotic dried treats such as strawberries, cranberries, cherries or blueberries. You can also vary the spices: try nutmeg, allspice, anise, ginger, mace or cardamom.

> 3 cups quick-cooking oats
> 1 teaspoon cinnamon
> 1/4 teaspoon cloves
> 3/4 cup chopped dates
> 3/4 cup dried apricots, chopped
> 1 cup apple butter
> 1 tablespoon sugar

Preheat the oven to 350° F. Mix the oats, cinnamon and cloves in a large bowl. Add the dates and apricots, then stir in the apple butter. Mix with a large spoon or your hands until all the ingredients are well blended and the oats are moistened with the apple butter.

Spread the mixture in an 8-by-13-inch nonstick pan and pat it down so you have an even layer covering the bottom of the pan. Sprinkle the sugar over the surface. Bake for 20 minutes.

Immediately cut into 2-inch squares but do not remove from the pan. Allow the bars to cool, then go over the cuts with a knife again. Remove the bars from the pan with a small spatula and store in a sealed container. They're even better on the second day.

24 2-inch bars

Candied Orange Peel

If you eat lots of oranges, as I do, you can save the peels and occasionally make up a batch of candied peel. I like to nibble on it like candy or add it to fruit breads, curries or fruit salads — any place I would use raisins. Cut oranges in quarters, peel and eat them out of hand, then place the peels in a plastic bag and collect them in your refrigerator. When you have a full bag, you're ready for this recipe.

> 8 cups orange peel
> 1 cup light Karo syrup
> 2 cups water
> 3 cups granulated sugar
> Additional granulated sugar (1 to 2 cups)

If the orange peels have a lot of white pith, scrape some of it off with a spoon. Thin peels do not need to be scraped. Put the orange peels in a large, heavy pot; cover with water, bring to a boil and simmer 15 minutes. Drain and repeat: cover the peel with fresh water, bring to a boil again, cook 15 minutes and drain. Slice the peels into ¼-inch-wide strips.

Place the syrup, water and sugar in a large, heavy pot and heat to dissolve the sugar. Stir in the orange peel and bring to a boil. Turn the heat down so the liquid boils very gently and cook, stirring occasionally, 1 hour.

Drain the peel in a colander and allow it to cool.

Cover a cookie sheet or large platter with foil or wax paper. When the orange peel is cool enough to handle, roll the pieces in a bowl of granulated sugar to coat lightly. Set them in a single layer on the cookie sheet and allow the peel to dry 2 to 3 days. Roll the pieces in sugar again and place in a container with a tight-fitting lid.

About 4 cups

Hawaiian Smoothie

This can be dessert, a breakfast treat or a snack anytime of day. You can make any amount, but blend it in small batches.

> 1 banana
> 1 cup orange juice or tropical fruit drink
> 2 cups fresh or frozen fruit of your choice — berries, melon, peaches, pineapple, oranges, whatever you have

Place the banana and juice in a blender and blend until smooth. Blend in the remaining fruit. Serve either as a thick drink or in bowls with a spoon.

2 servings

Maple-Glazed Fruit Bowls

Here's a combination that's equally delicious hot or cold — it's your choice.

> 3 oranges, peeled and sliced
> 3 kiwifruit, peeled and sliced
> 2 bananas, peeled and sliced
> 1/4 cup maple syrup
> 1/4 cup orange juice

Arrange the fruit slices in 4 heat-proof bowls. Mix the syrup and juice, and drizzle a little over each portion. When ready to serve, place the bowls on a broiler pan or cookie sheet and broil, 4 inches from the heat, 2 to 3 minutes. Or serve slightly chilled.

4 servings

Five-Fruit Curry

My passion for curry doesn't stop with the main course. The spices that make vegetables sparkle do wonders for fruit. If you keep your kitchen stocked with frozen, canned and dried fruits, you can whip up a dessert for company on a moment's notice. Here's one combination; you can invent lots more, and of course, you don't have to stop with five fruits.

> ½ cup orange juice or juice from the canned fruits
> ½ teaspoon curry powder
> ¼ teaspoon ground ginger or 1 tablespoon candied ginger, chopped
> 1 apple, peeled, cored and cut into bite-size pieces
> ½ cup raisins
> ½ cup dried apricots, cut into small pieces
> 1 cup sliced peaches, fresh or canned
> 1 cup pineapple chunks, fresh or canned

Heat the juice and spices in a saucepan large enough to hold all the fruits. Stir in the apple, raisins and apricots and cook gently, covered, until the dried fruits are plump — 5 to 10 minutes. Stir in the peaches and pineapple and heat through. Serve warm or chilled.

4 to 6 servings

Peaches and Raspberries

This simple, winning combination is at its best in summertime, but you can use frozen fruits off-season, too. All frozen fruits taste best when they are only partially thawed, with a few ice crystals left.

> 2 cups peaches, peeled and sliced
> 1 cup raspberries
> Sugar to taste

Place the peach slices in a glass bowl. Make a well in the center and spoon in the raspberries. If the fruits are very tart, sprinkle with a little sugar.

4 servings

Spiced Rhubarb and Oranges

I never liked rhubarb until I learned it doesn't need to be cooked to mush. Try it combined with oranges, raisins and spices.

    1 pound rhubarb
    3 cups water
    2 cups sugar
    1 teaspoon cinnamon
    ¼ teaspoon ground cloves
    1 cup golden raisins
    4 oranges, peeled and sliced
    Mint leaves for garnish (optional)

Wash the rhubarb, trim off the ends and slice the stalks into 1-inch pieces. Bring the water, sugar and spices to a boil in a large pot; add the rhubarb and the raisins and reduce the heat. Simmer until the rhubarb is tender when pierced with a fork, about 10 minutes. Drain off most of the liquid and stir in the orange slices. Transfer to a bowl and refrigerate. Serve chilled, garnished with mint leaves if desired.

4 to 6 servings

My Favorite Fruity Rice Pudding

It's hard to believe, but this fat-free rice pudding tastes just as good as the kind my mother made — maybe better. Like an Indian *kheer*, it's slightly soupy and full of fruit and spices. It's also very easy to make and quick if you use leftover rice.

    1 cup skim milk
    1 cup cooked brown rice
    ½ cup golden raisins
    ½ cup dried apricots, chopped
    ¼ teaspoon cinnamon
    Pinch ground cloves
    Pinch ground cardamom or the seeds from 4 cardamom pods (optional)

Warm the milk in a saucepan over low heat. Stir in the remaining ingredients, cover and cook very gently 15 to 20 minutes, stirring occasionally. Do not let the milk boil. The pudding is done when the fruits are plump and soft and most of the milk is absorbed.

Alternate cooking method: If you have an electric steamer, mix all of the ingredients in the rice bowl and steam 30 minutes.

3 to 4 servings

Appetizers and Snacks

Most commercially prepared "munchies" — chips, crackers, nuts, dips — are loaded with fat and have little nutritional value. But everyone loves to snack. Arm yourself with a repertoire of delicious and nutritious fat-free or very low fat munchies so you can snack to your heart's content.

Popcorn is a good fat-free snack as long as you don't add butter or oil. Sprinkle with seasoned salt or other spices and enjoy. Pretzels are lower in fat than other packaged snack foods, but they are also low in fiber and can't be eaten in unlimited quantities. Don't forget that old standby, raw vegetables. Keep a container of salad starter vegetables (page 252) on hand for spur-of-the-moment nibbling.

Here are some other ideas for low-fat appetizers and snack foods. They're good enough to serve to company.

Hummus

The traditional Middle Eastern spread is made with oil and high-fat sesame seeds. I think my low-fat version is every bit as good. Serve it with wedges of toasted pita bread or use it as a dip for raw vegetables.

> 2 cans chick peas, drained, or 3 cups cooked
> 1 onion, chopped
> 2 cloves garlic, minced
> 1 cup tomato puree
> ¼ cup lemon juice
> 2 teaspoons ground cumin
> ½ teaspoon paprika
> ¼ teaspoon cayenne or to taste
> Freshly ground black pepper to taste
> Cilantro or Italian parsley, chopped

Puree the chick peas, onion, garlic, tomato puree and lemon juice in a blender. Stir in the spices and season with black pepper to taste. Garnish with chopped cilantro or parsley.

About 3 cups

Chili Bean Dip

Serve this zesty dip with oil-free tortilla chips or raw vegetables.

> 1 can kidney beans, drained
> 2 tablespoons finely chopped jalapeño chiles, or to taste
> 1 tablespoon chili powder
> ¼ teaspoon cumin
> 1 tablespoon minced onion
> 1 tablespoon Italian parsley, chopped
> 1 tablespoon vinegar

Mash the ingredients together or puree them in a blender.

About 1½ cups

Snappy Bean Dip

Another bean dip — with a different accent.

> 1 can pinto or kidney beans, drained, or 2 cups cooked
> Juice of ½ lemon
> 2 tablespoons nonfat mayonnaise
> 1 teaspoon Worcestershire sauce
> 1 fresh or canned jalapeño pepper, seeded and chopped
> 3 green onions, sliced

Mash the ingredients together or puree them in a blender.

About 1½ cups

Chick Pea Dip or Dressing

This simple chick pea dip is good with fresh vegetables, as a dressing for a green salad or with lettuce and cucumber in pita bread.

> 1 can chick peas, drained
> ¼ cup bouillon (see page 187)
> 3 tablespoons lemon juice
> 2 cloves garlic
> 1 teaspoon paprika
> 1 teaspoon freshly ground black pepper or to taste

Puree all the ingredients in a blender. Add a little more bouillon if needed to give a smooth consistency to the dip or to make a slightly more liquid dressing.

About 1½ cups

Fake Guacamole

Unfortunately for Mexican food fans, avocados are excessively high in fat, and there's just no substitute for their taste and texture. This pea concoction doesn't taste anything like the real thing, but it has a pretty color and a nice flavor of its own.

> 3 cups frozen green peas, thawed
> 1 red onion, chopped
> 2 cloves garlic, minced
> 1 teaspoon cumin
> Pinch cayenne or to taste
> Freshly ground black pepper to taste

Puree all the ingredients in a blender. Use as a spread for toasted pita bread or as a dip, or roll in a flour tortilla with black beans and salsa for a low-fat burrito.

About 2 cups

Eggplant Caviar

Yet another good dip for raw vegetables or toasted pita bread triangles.

>*1 eggplant*
>*1 onion, chopped*
>*2 cloves garlic, minced*
>*3 tablespoons lemon juice*
>*¼ cup Italian parsley, chopped*

Roast the eggplant over a gas flame or under the broiler until the skin is charred and the eggplant is soft, about 10 minutes. Cool it and rub most of the skin off. Mash the eggplant pulp, put it in a strainer and press gently to drain off the liquid. Stir in the remaining ingredients. If a very smooth dip is desired, puree it in a blender.

About 2 cups

Far East Eggplant Spread

Eggplant doesn't have a strong flavor of its own, so it takes on the character of the seasonings you add. This spread tastes quite different from the preceding recipe.

>*1 eggplant*
>*1 tablespoon grated gingerroot*
>*2 cloves garlic, minced*
>*¼ cup cilantro leaves, chopped*
>*Pinch cayenne or to taste*
>*1 tablespoon rice wine vinegar*
>*1 tablespoon soy sauce*

Roast the eggplant over a gas flame or under a broiler until the skin is charred and the flesh is soft, about 10 minutes. Cool and remove most of the peel. Mash with the remaining ingredients or puree in a blender.

About 2 cups

Garlic-Parsley Spread

Toasted pita wedges are good with this simple spread, too.

> 1 cup Italian parsley, finely chopped
> 2 large cloves garlic, pressed (or use roasted garlic, page 306)
> ½ cup nonfat mayonnaise

Combine all the ingredients.

About 1 cup

Deviled Mushrooms

My deviled mushrooms are tasty enough for a party and simple enough for a quick snack.

> 1 pound mushrooms (sliced if large)
> ¼ cup Worcestershire sauce
> ¼ cup wine vinegar
> 2 tablespoons finely chopped onion
> 2 cloves garlic, minced
> ¼ teaspoon cayenne or to taste

Mix all the ingredients and marinate the mushrooms for at least 2 hours. Broil for 5 minutes. Serve with toasted pita bread or French bread.

4 to 6 servings

Herb-Garlic Cheese

If you yearn for those high-fat herb cheeses from the gourmet shop, try my yogurt cheese version. Sometimes I even fool myself. Use it as a dip with fresh vegetables, spread it on pita toasts or mix it with a little vinegar or lemon juice for a supreme salad dressing.

> 1 cup yogurt cheese (see page 313)
> 6 cloves roasted garlic, mashed, or 2 cloves plain garlic, minced
> ¼ cup chopped fresh herbs (oregano, marjoram, chives, whatever you wish)
> 1 tablespoon coarsely ground black pepper (optional)

Mix all the ingredients together and refrigerate, covered, for several hours or overnight. Keeps well for several days.

About 1 cup

Low-Fat Cup-of-Noodles

Those instant "cup-of-noodles" you see in the supermarket would be convenient as a quick snack or hot lunch to eat in your office, but they're loaded with fat (about 13 grams a cup). You can make your own low-fat version as easily as you make a cup of tea.

> *2 ounces Chinese curly noodles*
> *1 package instant cup-of-soup mix*
> *Boiling water*

Buy a package of Chinese curly noodles. The brand in my supermarket (in the Asian food section) has 3 "bricks" of noodles in a 10-ounce package. Then pick out a package of instant cup-of-soup mix in a flavor that has no more than 1 gram of fat, such as Lipton's Spring Vegetable.

Break half of one of the noodle bricks into a large coffee mug and add 1 packet of the soup mix. Fill the cup with boiling water (or water from an instant hot water tap), cover your cup and let it sit for about 5 minutes. Stir and enjoy!

1 serving

Toasted Tortilla Strips

When you toast tortillas in the oven, they aren't nearly as crisp as purchased chips, but they're fresh and aromatic. Serve them with salsa or bean dip, or as an accompaniment to chili.

> *8-ounce package fresh corn tortillas*
> *Salt to taste*
> *Chili powder to taste (optional)*

Preheat the oven to 350°F. Slice the tortillas in ½-by-2-inch strips. Arrange in a single layer on one or two cookie sheets lined with aluminum foil. Sprinkle with salt and chili powder if desired. Toast in the oven

10 to 15 minutes, checking frequently, until crisp but not burned. Serve warm or cool and store in a tightly sealed container.

About 3 cups

Guiltless Garlic Bread

Roasting garlic turns each clove into a buttery capsule that can be squeezed onto warm bread or toast. You won't even miss the fat.

> 1 whole head of garlic
> 1 loaf French bread

Preheat the oven to 400°F. Wrap the head of garlic in foil or place it in a small covered casserole and bake it for 45 minutes. Cut the loaf of French bread in half lengthwise and then into serving-size pieces. Toast the bread for a few minutes in the oven (400°F.). To serve, break the head of garlic into individual cloves, squeeze a clove with your fingers and spread the soft garlic onto pieces of the bread.

4 to 6 servings

Staples

This is a catch-all section of recipes for basic ingredients to have on hand in your pantry, refrigerator or freezer.

I think the spice mixes are essential. I would never be without a small container of harissa, and berbere is just about as indispensable.

Stock is not as critical because you can always use bouillon cubes, but if you keep a stock pot going, you can put lots of scraps to good use.

Tomato and chile sauces can be made in large quantities and frozen. The fresh salsas are always nice to have on hand, and I find lots of uses for yogurt cheese and roasted garlic.

Browse through these basic recipes and stock up!

Harissa (Moroccan-Style Hot Spice Blend)

If you've read this far, you know that a lot of my recipes use harissa. Remember, a little goes a long way! Stir in a tiny bit while you cook, or have diners mix a little into their own portion of any vegetable or bean dish. Be sure to caution anyone who is not familiar with harissa; I don't want you to lose a friend.

> 1 teaspoon caraway seed
> 2 tablespoons cayenne
> 1 tablespoon ground cumin
> 1 clove garlic
> ½ teaspoon salt
> ¼ cup nonfat Italian salad dressing

Put the dried spices in a blender and blend until the caraway is ground fine. Add the garlic and salad dressing and blend again. Store covered in the refrigerator. Very hot!

About ¼ cup

Berbere (Ethiopian Hot Spice Mix)

Berbere is not quite as fiery as harissa, but it's still a good idea to add a little at a time and taste as you go. Berbere is the perfect seasoning for lentils and just about any combination of beans and vegetables.

> 2 teaspoons cumin seed
> 1 teaspoon cardamom seed
> ½ teaspoon whole allspice
> 1 teaspoon fenugreek seed
> 1 teaspoon coriander seed
> 8 whole cloves
> 1 teaspoon black peppercorns
> 5 teaspoons red pepper flakes or crumbled dried red peppers
> 1 tablespoon grated fresh gingerroot or ½ teaspoon dried ginger
> 1 teaspoon turmeric
> 1 teaspoon salt
> 3 tablespoons sweet paprika
> ½ teaspoon cinnamon

Toast the seeds and whole cloves in a small frying pan for 2 minutes, stirring constantly. Grind the spices in a spice grinder. Mix in the remaining ingredients. Place in a tightly covered container and store in the refrigerator.

About ¼ cup

Fish Stock

When you have fish cleaned, ask the fishmonger to wrap the trimmings for you. It's worth making a pot of stock for future seafood soups. You can add the water you use to cook shrimp, or if you peel shrimp before cooking, simmer their shells in a cup or two of water, strain and add the liquid to the stock pot.

> 2 pounds white fish trimmings, heads, tails and bones
> 2 quarts water
> 1 cup dry white wine
> 1 onion, chopped
> 2 carrots, chopped
> 2 stalks celery, chopped
> 1 bay leaf
> Several sprigs fresh thyme or ½ teaspoon dried
> 10 whole peppercorns

Bring all the ingredients to a boil and simmer 1 hour. Strain, cool and refrigerate or freeze.

About 2 quarts

Vegetable Stock

Use vegetable stock in place of water in any recipe.

> 3 quarts water
> 4 onions, chopped
> 2 potatoes, chopped
> 4 carrots, sliced
> 4 stalks celery, sliced
> 2 bay leaves
> 10 peppercorns
> Optional:
>   Any other vegetable scraps
>   Parsley or any other fresh herbs, as desired

Bring the water to a boil; add all the ingredients and simmer 1 hour or more. Strain. Use within 1 week or freeze.

About 3 quarts

Browned Flour

If you have recipes that use flour browned in fat to thicken sauces, try substituting the fat-free, oven-browned version. To use, mix a little of the browned flour in a small amount of cold water or stock and stir into the sauce or soup as it cooks. Use ¼ cup flour in ¼ to ½ cup liquid to thicken a good-sized pot of gumbo or vegetable stew.

> *1 to 2 cups flour*

Preheat the oven to 325° F. Spread the flour on a nonstick cookie sheet and bake in the oven 1 hour. Store in a tightly covered container and use for thickening soups, gumbos and stews.

1 to 2 cups

Chunky Tomato Sauce

This sauce is good on grains or pasta, or you can use it in any recipe that calls for tomato sauce. If you have a bumper crop of fresh tomatoes, by all means use them in this recipe.

> 2 onions, chopped
> 2 carrots, chopped
> 2 stalks celery, chopped
> 2 cloves garlic, minced
> 2 cans (29 ounces each) plum tomatoes, chopped
> 2 tablespoons fresh oregano or 2 teaspoons dried
> ¼ cup fresh basil leaves, chopped
> ¼ cup Italian parsley, chopped

Cook the onion, carrots, celery and garlic in a little of the juice from the tomatoes until softened, about 10 minutes. Add the tomatoes and oregano and cook 15 to 20 minutes. Stir in the basil and parsley.

About 6 cups

Tomato Sauce

Here's an even quicker tomato sauce that's still very good.

>   1 large onion, chopped
>   4 cloves garlic, minced or pressed
>   2 cans (28 ounces each) cans tomato sauce (I use Hunt's)
>   1 tablespoon fresh oregano or 1 teaspoon dried
>   1 bay leaf

Combine all the ingredients in a pot and bring to a boil. Simmer, covered, 30 minutes, stirring occasionally. If a thicker sauce is desired, remove the cover and simmer 5 to 10 minutes longer.

About 6 cups

Mexican Tomato Sauce

A basic tomato sauce with a south-of-the-border accent.

>   1 onion, chopped
>   3 cloves garlic, chopped
>   1 green pepper, chopped
>   1/4 cup dry red wine or bouillon
>   1 can (28 ounces) plum tomatoes, chopped
>   1 teaspoon chili powder
>   1 teaspoon cumin
>   1/4 teaspoon cayenne or to taste
>   2 tablespoons lemon juice
>   1/4 cup cilantro or Italian parsley, chopped
>   Freshly ground black pepper

Cook the onion, garlic and green pepper in the wine or bouillon until softened, about 10 minutes. Add the tomatoes and spices and cook 10 minutes. Stir in the lemon juice and cilantro and season with pepper to taste.

About 3 cups

Red Chile Sauce

Your own chile sauce takes the place of chili powder. Stir it into beans or use it in any of the vegetable chili recipes.

> 10 dried red New Mexican chiles (see page 138)
> 1 onion, chopped
> 2 cloves garlic, minced
> 1 teaspoon cumin
> 3 cups bouillon (see page 187)

Preheat the oven to 200°F. and toast the chiles 5 minutes. Remove the stems and seeds and tear the chile pods into pieces. Place the chiles, onion, garlic, cumin and 1 cup of the bouillon in a blender and puree until smooth. Pour the mixture into a saucepan; add the remaining bouillon, bring to a boil and simmer 1 hour.

About 3 cups

Fresh Salsa

Salsas can be as tame or as spicy as you like. These three recipes are my favorites, but you can combine the basic vegetables in any proportion you like. Serve salsa as a dip with oil-free tortilla chips or mix it with black beans or kidney beans for a delicious, simple chili.

> 4 ripe tomatoes, chopped
> 2 jalapeño chiles, seeded and chopped
> 1 red onion, chopped
> 1 clove garlic, minced
> ¼ cup cilantro, chopped
> 1 tablespoon lime or lemon juice
> 1 teaspoon cumin

Combine all the ingredients and let the flavors blend for at least 1 hour before serving. Keeps well; refrigerate in a covered container.

About 2 cups

Tomatillo Salsa

Serve tomatillo salsa with chips at room temperature or chilled, or stir it into a pot of cooked beans for a tasty green chili.

20 tomatillos (greenhusk tomatoes)
1 onion, chopped
2 cloves garlic, minced
1 jalapeño chile, seeded and minced
½ cup bouillon (see page 187)
1 teaspoon ground coriander
¼ cup cilantro leaves, chopped

Remove the papery husks and cut the tomatillos into quarters. Cook them with the onion, garlic, chile and ground coriander in the bouillon 15 to 20 minutes. Stir in the cilantro.

About 2 cups

Green Chile Salsa

This salsa is great with broiled fish and also makes a good green chili. I love it with black beans.

1 onion, chopped
4 cloves garlic
1 jalapeño pepper, seeded and minced
1 teaspoon cumin
½ cup bouillon (see page 187)
6 mild green chiles, roasted, peeled, seeded and chopped, or 2 cans (4 ounces each) chopped green chiles (see page 138)
1 cup cilantro leaves, chopped

Simmer the onion, garlic, jalapeño pepper and cumin in the stock 10 minutes, or until the onions are soft. Stir in the green chiles and cilantro.

About 2 cups

Roasted Garlic

Roasted garlic is buttery-soft and mild. Squeeze it onto warm French bread or use in salad dressings, soups or any recipe where a mild garlic flavor is desired.

1 or more whole heads of garlic, unpeeled

Preheat the oven to 400°F. Place the garlic heads in a covered oven-proof dish and bake 45 minutes. Cool, break apart the cloves, and squeeze with your fingers. You can store roasted garlic in your refrigerator, covered, for several days.

As much as you want

Yogurt Cheese

Yogurt cheese can be used as a fat-free substitute in salads and appetizers that would use feta, goat cheese or any other tangy cheese. I like to mix in garlic and herbs or ground black pepper (see page 304).

1 pint (or more) plain nonfat yogurt

Line a colander with four paper towels and pour in the yogurt. Cover with another paper towel and place the colander in a pan. Let the yogurt sit at room temperature for 24 hours. Discard the liquid and remove the "cheese" from the paper towels. Store in the refrigerator.

About 1 cup

Glossary of Unusual Ingredients

Cellophane noodles: Thread-like, almost transparent noodles found in Asian groceries or the Asian section of your supermarket. They cook quickly and have a slightly crunchy texture.

Chiles, dried New Mexican or ancho: The large, dark red chiles that are used to make sauces and "authentic" chili. Usually mild, but sometimes they are a little hot. Check the produce department of your supermarket or find them in Hispanic markets. Refer to A Pepper Primer, page 138.

Cilantro: Also known as Chinese parsley or fresh coriander. Find it in Asian or Hispanic groceries and many supermarkets. It looks a lot like Italian parsley, so you may need to taste a leaf to avoid a mix-up. Most recipes call for chopped cilantro leaves. You can also use the stems and washed roots to flavor soup stock.

Dashi: A Japanese broth made with seaweed and fish. You can buy instant dashi in Asian markets and many supermarkets. Good to use as stock in any fish soup.

Fish sauce: A thin, salty liquid made from shrimp or anchovies, used in Thai and Vietnamese cooking. Asian groceries carry several brands. This is an acquired taste; use very small amounts at first.

Galanga: Looks like gingerroot, but with its own distinctive flavor; used in southeast Asian cooking to flavor soups and stocks. My Asian grocery carries frozen sliced galanga; if you live in a large city, you may be able to buy it fresh. Don't bother with dried galanga; if you can't find fresh or frozen, just leave it out of the recipe.

Kaffir lime leaves: Fresh or dried leaves of an aromatic citrus tree, sometimes available in Asian groceries. They add a wonderful fragrance to soups and curries. If you can't find them, substitute a little grated lime rind.

Lemon grass: A tough grass with a lemony flavor and fragrance. Used in southeast Asian cooking to flavor soups and sauces. Look for fresh lemon grass in Asian markets; dried lemon grass is tasteless. Only the bottom 6 inches or so of the stalk is used. Cut off the root end and pound the stalk or slice it into ¼-inch pieces. You can substitute grated lemon rind, but it's not the same.

Mango chutney: A sweet, spicy preserve made with mangoes, raisins and tamarind, traditionally served with curry. The gourmet section of your supermarket probably has several brands. You can make your own chutneys from fresh or canned fruits; see pages 294 to 295.

Nori: The dried seaweed used to wrap sushi; available in sheets in Asian markets. The other kinds of dried seaweed you will find there are good for flavoring fish soups.

Ginger, pickled: Slivers of pickled gingerroot served with sushi and other Japanese specialties; available in jars in Asian markets and some supermarkets. Pickled ginger is neither sweet nor hot, but it has a distinctive bite of its own. If you like it with sushi, try it as an accompaniment to other fish or spicy foods.

Ginger, candied: Candied or crystallized ginger can be nibbled like candy or chopped and added to fruit desserts or salads. I usually find it in the gourmet or Asian sections of the supermarket and sometimes in the produce section. You can buy it in large packages, usually at a much lower price than elsewhere, in Asian grocery stores.

Rice wine vinegar: A light vinegar that tastes very different from other vinegars. Use it to dress a salad all by itself. Especially good with bok choy or Chinese cabbage. In the Asian food section of your supermarket.

Soba and other Asian noodles: Soba are Japanese noodles made with buckwheat flour. These and dozens of other kinds of noodles are available in Asian groceries and, increasingly, in supermarkets. Try both dried and fresh noodles. If there are no cooking directions on the package, just cook them like spaghetti and check every few minutes for tenderness.

Star anise: The flower-shaped whole pods impart their anise flavor to soup or cooking liquid and are removed before serving. Ground star anise is one of the ingredients in Chinese five-spice powder (see page 63).

Surimi: Shredded fish shaped and flavored to resemble crab or lobster. See page 172.

Tamarind: The bean-shaped fruit of a tropical tree, with a citrusy pulp and large seeds. Available in Asian markets in compressed, seedless blocks. Use it in sauces, chutneys and anywhere you'd like an unusual sweet-tart touch. If you can't get tamarind, substitute lemon or lime juice.

Tomatillo: A small, green tomato-like fruit with a papery husk. In Hispanic groceries and sometimes in the specialty produce section of the supermarket. Remove the husks; quarter the tomatillos and simmer in a little stock.

Wasabi: "Japanese horseradish." A green powder that comes in small cans; you add water to make a thick paste. Essential with sushi and can be used in sauces or as a seasoning for other fish dishes. Start with a little bit; it's "hot," not like chile peppers, but like a very powerful horseradish.

Notes

I have cited a variety of studies and articles throughout this book. The following references are provided in case you wish to do additional research or share my sources of information with your physician.

1. *American Journal of Clinical Nutrition*, 1984, vol. 39, pp. 35–44.
2. Mirkin, Gabe, and Marshall Hoffman, *The Sportsmedicine Book*, Little Brown, 1979.
3. *Neuroscience and Biobehavioral Reviews*, 1992, vol. 16, pp. 585–596; *American Journal of Clinical Nutrition*, 1992, vol. 56, pp. 616–622.
4. *American Journal of Clinical Nutrition*, 1992, vol. 56, pp. 887–894.
5. *New England Journal of Medicine*, 1991, vol. 324, pp. 1839–1844.
6. *Lancet*, 1990, vol. 336, pp. 129–133.
7. *Circulation*, 1992, vol. 86, pp. 1046–1060.
8. *British Medical Journal*, 1990, vol. 301, pp. 309–313; *Archives of Internal Medicine*, 1992, vol. 152, pp. 1490–1500.
9. *Hypertension*, 1991, vol. 18 (suppl. 1), pp. 115–120; *New York Times*, December 31, 1991, p. C-1; *Klin Wochenschrift*, 1990, vol. 68, pp. 664–668, and vol. 69 (suppl.), pp. 51–57.
10. *Lancet*, 1992, vol. 340, pp. 925–929.
11. *Journal of the National Cancer Institute*, 1990, vol. 82, pp. 129–134; *American Journal of Clinical Nutrition*, 1990, vol. 51, p. 371.
12. *Journal of the American Medical Association*, 1992, vol. 268, pp. 2037–2044.
13. *Journal of the National Cancer Institute*, 1992, vol. 84, pp. 47–51.
14. *Prevention* magazine, May 1993, pp. 38–46.
15. *New England Journal of Medicine*, 1991, vol. 324, pp. 1839–1844.
16. *Journal of the American Medical Association*, 1992, vol. 268, pp. 2037–2044.
17. *Journal of Family Practice*, 1991, vol. 33, pp. 249–254; *Journal of the American Medical Association*, 1991, vol. 265, pp. 3285–3291, *British Medical Journal*, 1991, vol. 303, pp. 953–957.
18. *American Journal of Clinical Nutrition*, 1992, vol. 55, pp. 385–394.
19. *Canadian Medical Association Journal*, 1992, vol. 147, pp. 900.
20. *New England Journal of Medicine*, 1994, vol. 330, pp. 1029–1035.
21. *Scottish Medical Journal*, 1992, vol. 37, pp. 49–52; *Journal of the American College of Nutrition*, 1992, vol. 11, pp. 139–144; *Critical Reviews in Food Science and Nutrition*, 1992, vol. 32, pp. 33–57.

22. *American Journal of Clinical Nutrition*, 1991, vol. 53 (suppl.), pp. 314S–321S.

23. *Journal of the National Cancer Institute*, 1993, vol. 85, pp. 1571–1579.

24. *Circulation*, 1992, vol. 86, pp. 803–811.

25. *Annals of Internal Medicine*, 1991, vol. 115, pp. 505–512.

26. *Gastroenterology*, 1991, vol. 101, pp. 977–990.

27. *American Journal of Clinical Nutrition*, 1991, vol. 53, pp. 106–111; *Obstetrics and Gynecology*, 1983, vol. 61, pp. 456–462.

28. *Washingtonian* magazine, February 1992, pp. 70–79.

29. *Cardiovascular Reviews and Reports*, May 1986, vol. 7, pp. 461–472.

30. *Journal of the Federation of American Societies of Experimental Biology*, 1992, vol. 6, p. 2600.

31. *Journal of Nutritional Science and Vitaminology*, 1990, vol. 36 (suppl.), pp. 81S–86S; *The Physician and Sportsmedicine*, 1991, vol. 19, pp. 19–22.

32. *Journal of the American Medical Association*, 1992, vol. 267, pp. 3317–3325.

33. *Journal of the American Dietetic Association*, 1991, vol. 91, pp. 820–827.

34. *Archives of Internal Medicine*, 1992, vol. 152, pp. 1416–1424; and 1993, vol. 153, p. 125.

35. *Journal of the Federation of American Societies of Experimental Biology*, 1990, vol. 4, pp. 2652–2660.

36. Deutsch, Ronald, *Realities of Nutrition*, Bull Publishing Company, 1976, p. 9.

37. *New England Journal of Medicine*, 1987, vol. 316, p. 1174; *Journal of the American Medical Association*, 1988, vol. 260, p. 652; *World Health Organization Statistical Annual*, 1990, p. 40.

38. *New England Journal of Medicine*, 1990, vol. 323, p. 759.

39. *Nutrition Action Health Letter*, May 1991, p. 4.

40. Exercise Guidelines announced by the President's Council on Physical Fitness, the American College of Sports Medicine and CDC, July 1993.

41. *Acta Physiologica Scandanavica*, 1960, vol. 48, pp. 448–453.

42. *New England Journal of Medicine*, 1994, vol. 330, pp. 1776–1781; *American Journal of Clinical Nutrition*, 1994, vol. 59 (suppl.), pp. 1238S–1241S.

43. *New England Journal of Medicine*, 1989, vol. 321, pp. 929–933.

44. *Circulation*, 1994, vol. 89, pp. 969–974.

45. *Digestive Diseases and Sciences*, 1993, vol. 38, pp. 2262–2266.

Index

cereals, 18
 granola, 52
cheeses, "light" or "low fat," 55–56
chicken, 8, 15, 16, 56, 122
chili powder, 63
Chinese ingredients, 85
Chinese parsley (cilantro), 65–66
chives, 65
cholesterol (blood), 4, 17, 129
 cheating on fatty foods and, 10
 cholesterol consumption and, 33, 36, 56- 57
 drugs in lowering of, 7, 22–23
 exercise and, 7–8
 fat consumption and, 15, 21, 23–24, 33, 35
 fiber and, 15–16, 53, 118
 measuring of, 19, 129
 nibbling and, 114
 oat bran and, 50–51
 omega-3's and, 47
 reducing only saturated fat and, 8, 34–35, 119
 small restrictions in fat intake and, 33, 35
 soybeans and, 51, 120
 substituting poultry for meat and, 8
 tropical oils and, 47
 very low levels of, 24–25, 130
 vitamin C and, 38–39
 wine and, 52–53
 see also HDL cholesterol; LDL cholesterol
cholesterol (dietary), 32, 33, 35–36
 blood cholesterol and, 33, 36, 56–57
 in shellfish, 122
cilantro, 65
Circulation, 24
cirrhosis, 53
citrus juice, 68
clam juice, 68
clenbutarol, 99–100
clotting, 19, 47, 52, 128–129
coconut oil, 45, 47
colon cancer, 17, 28, 30, 46, 118
condiments, 78
 see also spices and seasonings
constipation, 16, 17, 53, 118
contrast, as flavor full principle, 60–61
cookies, 10
cooking liquids, 67–68
cooking methods, low-fat, 68–69
cooling down, after exercise, 127
coriander, fresh (cilantro), 65–66
cortisone-type injections, 100
cross-country ski machines, 107
curry powder, 63

dairy products, 9, 51
 see also milk; yogurt
dancing, aerobic, 106
Davis, Adelle, 52
depression, 24, 130
diabetes, 3, 13, 17, 27–28, 118
diet pills, 115

diets, 4
 commercial programs and, 41–42
 fad, 33, 41–42
 liquid, 117
 metabolic rate and, 114–115
 misconceptions about, 32–42
 restricted-calorie, 5, 9, 33–34, 115
 see also low-fat diet
diglycerides, 48–49, 120
dill, 66
dinner, 80–81
diuretics, 27
Doctor's Quick Weight Loss Diet, 41
Drinking Man's Diet, 41
drugs:
 cholesterol-lowering, 7, 22–23
 for muscle injuries, 99–100

eating out, 82, 87
eggs, 15, 45, 51, 56–57
endorphins, 91
estrogen, 29, 130–131
ethnic cuisines, 10, 61–62
ethnic grocery stores, 85–86
exercise, 27, 90–112, 124–128
 aerobic dancing, 106
 alternating sports in, 93–94
 amount of, 92–93
 beneficial effects of, 13
 best time for, 99
 bicycling, 109
 buying equipment for, 112
 cholesterol level and, 7–8
 choosing sports for, 103–112
 cooling down after, 127
 cross-country ski machines, 107
 duration of, 96–97
 after eating, 82, 99
 frequency of, 125–126
 good feelings as result of, 91
 "hard-easy principle" in, 92, 125–126
 injuries and, 8, 92, 96, 99–100, 126, 127
 intensity of, 94–96, 127–128
 jogging and running, 108, 127
 jogging on mini-trampoline, 106
 metabolism and, 5, 95, 115
 muscle soreness after, 96, 97
 and precautions for older people, 100–102, 126
 pulse rate and, 95–96, 127–128
 racquetball, handball or squash, 111
 rowing machines, 107
 setting goals for, 124–125
 skating or rollerblading, 110–111
 stair-steppers, 107
 starting program of, 92–94, 98–99
 stationary bicycles, 105, 125
 step aerobics, 106
 stress and recover method in, 92, 125
 stretching and, 127

metabolism, 14
  dieting and, 114–115
  after eating, 81–82, 114
  exercise and, 5, 95, 115
milk, 15
  low-fat, 57
  skim, 9, 12, 15, 57, 74, 76
millet, 71–72
minerals, 9
mini-trampolines, jogging on, 106
Mirkin Report, 10
monoglycerides, 48–49, 120
monounsaturated fats, 45, 46
muscles, 27, 31
  aging and, 100–102
  cooling down and, 127
  injuries to, 92, 96, 99–100, 126, 127
  maximum heart rate and, 128
  soreness of, 96, 97
  warming up, 98–99, 126–127
  weight loss and, 34

National Cancer Institute, 124
New England Journal of Medicine, 34, 56
19 Meals for Dr. Gabe rule, 10, 15, 82, 88
"no-cholesterol" foods, 35–36
Nutrition Action Health Letter, 56
nuts, 15, 46, 51

oat bran, 50–51, 121
oats, cooking, 71–72
oils, 9, 15, 45, 119
  spray, 119
  tropical, 45, 47
older people:
  exercise precautions for, 100–102, 126
  supplements for, 40
Olestra, 48
olive oil, 20, 43, 46
olives, 46
omega-3 polyunsaturated fats, 45, 46–47, 77
oregano, 66
Ornish, Dean, 18
osteoporosis, 40, 102, 111, 113, 130–131
overweight, 4, 17, 30–31
  diabetes and, 27, 28

palm kernel oil, 45, 47
palm oil, 45, 47
Pam, 119
pancreas, 51–52
pancreatic cancer, 24
parsley, 66
  Chinese (cilantro), 65–66
pasta, 9, 15, 16, 71, 77
peas, split, 71
peppers, 62–63
"percent fat free" claims, 54–55
phytochemicals, 16, 40–41
plaques, 4, 16, 18, 19, 20, 23, 52

blood pressure and, 26, 27
polydextrose, 48
polyunsaturated fats, 29, 45–46
  omega-3, 45, 46–47, 77
potatoes, 12, 16
poultry, 9, 15, 16, 56, 122
  substituting for meat, 8
pregnancy, 53
Prevention, 32
Pritikin, Nathan, 9
produce stands, 86
prolactin, 29
prostate cancer, 17, 28, 29, 46
proteins:
  amino acids in, 113–114
  calories in, 12
  converted to body fat, 13
  diets high in, 41
  need for, 113
pulse rate, exercise and, 95–96, 127–128

quinoa, cooking, 71–72

racquetball, 111
recipes, adapting for low-fat diet, 89
recovery period, after exercise, 92, 97
recumbent stationary bicycles, 105, 125
red pepper, 62–63
restaurant meals, 82, 87
resveratrol, 52
rice, 16, 114
  brown, cooking, 71–72
  white vs. brown, 16
rice cookers, 71–72
RICE treatment, 99
Rich, Diana, 10
roasting, 69
rollerblading, 110–111
rosemary, 66
rowing machines, 107
running, 108, 127
  on treadmill, 109

salad dressings, with artificial fats, 48
salt, 13, 26–27
saturated fats, 8, 29, 45
  restricting only intake of, 8, 33, 34–35, 119
  in tropical oils, 47
Scarsdale Diet, 41
seafood, 15, 74, 76, 77, 78, 122
  see also fish
seasonings. *See* spices and seasonings
seeds, 15, 46
selenium, 38–39
serving size, on food labels, 48, 54, 83
Seventh-Day Adventists, 51
shopping, low-fat, 83–86
  at ethnic grocery stores, 85–86
  at health food stores, 86
  making list for, 85

Recipe Index

Trial Offer for New Subscribers to *The Mirkin Report*

It's no secret that those who eat right and exercise regularly have a better chance for survival. They need less medical care, have more energy, and enjoy life to the fullest. The *Mirkin Report* helps you achieve and maintain a healthy lifestyle. Each month it brings you the latest medical breakthroughs and lots of helpful articles on nutrition, sexuality, and fitness. Every issue has a page of low-fat recipes.

I review the world's medical and scientific literature and give you the news that helps you stay fit and healthy. A one-year subscription is $39.95 (Maryland residents add $2.00 sales tax) for twelve monthly issues. With each new one-year subscription I will also send you my popular carry-along 20 Gram Diet and unique Fat Gram Counter that helps you keep a daily record of fat consumed. You may order a three-month trial subscription for only $4.95. With the *Mirkin Report* you can stay informed, slim, and healthy.

— *Dr. Gabe Mirkin*

For three months of the *Mirkin Report* please send $4.95 ($5.75 in Canada; overseas $6.95) to: *The Mirkin Report*, Fat Free Clinic, 5618 Shields Drive, Bethesda, MD 20817. Maryland residents add $.25 sales tax.